35 Practical Ways To Improve Your Health

A Common Sense Approach For Wholesome Living

35 Practical Ways To Improve Your HEALTH

A Common Sense Approach For Wholesome Living

Reid E. Lassonde

REAL-LIFE PUBLICATIONS
Minneapolis, Minnesota

REAL-LIFE PUBLICATIONS
8124 33rd Place North
Minneapolis, Minnesota 55427-1921

Copyright© 1992 by Reid E. Lassonde

All rights reserved. No part of this book may be reproduced or transmitted in any manner whatsoever without written permission from the author, except to quote brief passages in connection with reviews for a magazine, newspaper, or broadcast.

Cover Design: Reid E. Lassonde and Ronald Putt

Front Cover Art: Original pastel drawing, "Path to Enlightenment," 18" x 24", 1989, by Mary Fran Koppa and Copyright© 1992 by Reid E. Lassonde

Illustrations: Ronald Putt

Back Cover Photograph: Mary T.

Typesetting/Layout: Renee Putt
                      Graphics II
                      8034 Holden Road
                      Stevensville, Michigan 49127
                      Tel: (616) 422-1066
                      (Ronald and my twin sister Renee Putt—owners and operators)

First printing 1992
Printed and bound in the United States of America

Publisher's Cataloging in Publication
(Prepared by Quality Books Inc.)

Lassonde, Reid E., 1949-
    35 practical ways to improve your health : a common sense approach for wholesome living / Reid E. Lassonde.
    p. cm.
    Includes bibliographical references and index.
    Pre-assigned LCCN: 91-68336
    ISBN 0-9631846-7-9
    1. Nutrition. 2. Health.   I. Title. II. Title: Thirty-five practical ways to improve your health.

RA784.L3 1992   613
                                QBI92-428

Dedication

This book is respectfully dedicated to the following people who have directed and influenced me on my pursuit of a healthier body:

To the very fine Doctor Bernard Jensen who was my teacher during three intensive training sessions that I attended in San Diego and Escondido, California and Toronto, Ontario. Much of the information presented here is from knowledge and practical research that Dr. Jensen has generously shared through his lectures, books, tapes, and videos. He has treated more than 350,000 patients within the last 60 years.

His leadership in the advancement of nutrition and better health across this country is invaluable. To learn more about this remarkable man and his many contributions to humanity, be sure and read his book entitled *Nature Has a Remedy*.

All of Dr. Jensen's work (his writings, seminars, cassettes, etc.) is copyrighted. The author has signed an agreement with him that grants special permission to use his material throughout this book.

To Doctor Carey Reams who identified the vital functions of the liver and its important interrelationship with distilled water, along with many other key health ideas.

To Doctor Joseph Manthei who interpreted and simplified the knowledge that Dr. Reams taught him, besides expanding upon it.

To my friend and mentor, Doctor Gary Johnson, who patiently answered my unending stream of questions and helped motivate me to gain other knowledge.

To my mother, Elvina, who introduced me to nutrition in 1955, long before most people could even spell the word.

To my father, Ernest, who taught me how to "take the initiative."

To my friend, Beverly Verpaelst, for showing the value of the thymus gland.

Acknowledgements

Special thanks to Eunice, Debbie, Larry, Joan, Gayanne, Tony, and Mary Fran for their suggestions and help in the production of the following text.

This book was written, designed, edited, and published by the author. I humbly and gratefully acknowledge my Creator for the inspiration and guidance he gave me to complete this task:

> *And You called me, without using Your voice;*
> *And You touched me, without using Your fingers;*
> *And You supported me, without using Your arms;*
> *And You loved me, because that is what You are.*

Table of Contents

Introduction

Prologue

Chapter	Page
1. Alfalfa Tablets	15
2. All Spices & Herbs (ASH)	17
3. Aloe Vera	19
4. Bee Pollen	21
5. Belief In Someone Higher Than You	25
6. Blackstrap Molasses	27
7. Cayenne Pepper	29
8. Change Your Attitude	31
9. Chlorophyll	35
10. Cleanse Your Colon	37
11. Digestive Aids	45
12. Distilled Water	47
13. Exercise	51
14. Flaxseed	53
15. Herbal Teas	57
16. Iodine	61
17. Learn To Love	63
18. Liquid Minerals	67
19. Min-Col	71
20. Niacin Flush	77
21. Onion Soup	79
22. Potato Peeling Broth	81
23. Rainbow-Colored Salads	83
24. Raw Goat's Milk	85
25. Raw, Whole, & Pure	89
26. Rest	93
27. Rhythm	95
28. Rice Bran Syrup	97
29. Skin Brushing	99

Table of Contents

Chapter	Page
30. Spinal Adjustments	101
31. Tahini (Sesame Seed Butter)	103
32. Thump Your Thymus	105
33. Unclean Meats	109
34. Vitamin "E" & Lecithin	111
35. Wheat & Milk Allergies	113
Happy and Healthy, Naturally...	117
Epilogue: The Healing Crisis	123
Recommended Vendor List	125
Bibliography	129
Index	131

Introduction

If you are reading this book, it is probably fair to assume that you have an interest in maintaining or raising your present level of health. You may already be in good health, or perhaps you have recently noticed a decline in your energy or overall well-being. Maybe you just know that something isn't right. Regardless, no one has to tell you that something is wrong; you are much more in tune with your body than anyone else.

If your health isn't at the level you desire, what value, then, would you place on it? Perhaps you would say that your most valuable possession is the love of your family or friends. You might even say your freedom, or your job, or the money you receive from the toils of your hard labor. Your responses probably would be as diverse as people themselves.

Whatever, I believe they would all be wrong unless you answered that the most important possession you own is your health! If you think about it, without good health you could not enjoy or even support your spouse or family. And if you are sick, what value would money have if you were too unhealthy to appreciate the material goods that it can buy anyway?

Ask someone who is terminally ill what truly matters in this world! If they could make a choice between a million dollars or being well again, is there any doubt in your mind which one they would pick? Even a fortune in money can pale in comparison to the joy of living that a vibrant, healthy body would once again provide. The adage, you never realize what you have until you lose it, could not be more appropriate.

The following 35 chapters have been written with you in mind—to help you regain or improve your health. They have been prepared in an easy-to-understand format and were selected because they also can be easily incorporated into your daily living, and are inexpensive. I listed them alphabetically for reference purposes.

Several of them are based on biblical scriptures that have influenced and shaped my understanding of what constitutes good health. It is not my intent nor wish to convert anyone to my personal religious beliefs. Still, I felt it was important to include those verses that have taught me how to live better in harmony with nature and my Creator. You can then decide for yourself how valuable they are. This book represents my understanding of the truth; it does not have to be yours.

While it would be very time consuming and unrealistic for you to follow all the health ideas presented here, select those that fit your lifestyle, and leave the rest for later. As with all things, nothing is ever guaranteed. However, you should notice an improvement in your health by using any one or all 35 of these suggestions.

That improvement could occur in any of the following ways:

- You notice that your energy level is higher.
- People comment that you look better.
- Your skin color becomes healthier.
- There is a change in the amount of pain you feel.
- You are more positive about life in general.
- There is a reduction in the severity of your headaches or they stop altogether.
- You can do activities again that you could not do before.
- You notice an improvement in your allergies.
- You just plain "feel" better.

Whatever the changes you notice, celebrate and enjoy them, for you deserve all the best that healthful living can bring!

Prologue

This publication contains a personal listing of the products or practices that I believe can be used to improve your health. I also have included my recommended vendors, with their prices, at the back of the book to help guide you when making your purchases. Keep in mind the figures I am using are only an approximation of the actual costs involved; they will vary by state, location, vendor and are subject to change. They do not include any additional shipping or handling fees, where appropriate, or any applicable taxes. Always compare products or services before you buy.

To be sure that the maximum benefit is received from these recommendations, it would be advisable for you (although not an absolute requirement) to complete a several day, one week, or even longer cleansing program before using this information. The cleansing is invaluable because it prepares the body for any major changes that are to come in your diet or lifestyle. See Chapter 10 for more information on this important topic.

Warning — Disclaimer

None of the information contained in this book is intended in any way to supersede or replace the direction or guidance of your personal medical physician. No attempt has been made to diagnose or name any diseases and it must not be construed otherwise. Only a licensed doctor may diagnose or name diseases.

The author will not assume responsibility for the interpretations or actions of others who follow any of the suggestions as outlined in the ensuing chapters. Check with your doctor first if you have any concerns or questions.

No two people are alike, and we all react differently when changes are made in the foods we eat or in our belief systems. If anything recommended here causes you distress, discontinue its use immediately. Select only those nutrients, supplements, and techniques that feel right for you. Learn to listen to your body.

Caution: In some instances, I have noted the type and quantity of supplements I personally take. Note that the portions mentioned apply to adults only. Always use good judgement and smaller amounts if you are feeding them to children.

CHAPTER 1
Alfalfa Tablets

Alfalfa is one of nature's most nutritious plants. Translated, its name means the "father of all foods." It has a root system that can reach over a hundred feet deep into the ground. Because of this, alfalfa is very high in a variety of essential minerals that the body needs. Here is a list of the most important ones:

>aluminum
>calcium
>chlorine
>iron
>magnesium
>phosphorus
>potassium
>silicon
>sodium
>sulphur
>trace minerals

It contains vitamins A, B-complex, C, D, E, K (necessary for blood clotting), U (for peptic ulcers), and chlorophyll (see Chapter 9), and a natural fluoride that strengthens the teeth. Eight essential digestive enzymes and eight essential amino acids also are present in alfalfa.[1]

The eight essential amino acids must come from foods in our diet, as the body cannot produce them on its own (see Chapters 4, 14, & 25). Their names are isoleucine, leucine, lysine, methionine, phenylalanine, threonine, tryptophan, and valine.[2] They help support the body in various ways: phenylalanine is an anti-depressant, methionine interacts with the essential fatty acids (see Chapters 4, 14, 25, & 34),

---

[1]Penny C. Royal, *Herbally Yours*, 3rd ed. (Provo, Utah: Sound Nutrition, 1982), p. 14.
[2]Udo Erasmus, *Fats and Oils* (Vancouver, British Columbia: Alive Books, 1986), p. 264.

lysine is used to fight viruses and tryptophan is a sleep aid.[3]

Because of its high nutrient content, it has been used as a tablet supplement for many years. My mother was using Nutrilite® alfalfa tablets back in 1955, and I have taken them since I was a child.

The colon requires sodium, magnesium, and potassium to operate healthily[4] (see Chapter 10). Alfalfa has all three available in a plentiful supply.

It also tones and firms up the muscles of the colon wall as it contributes bulk throughout the elimination system. The added fiber helps rebuild the bowel sufficiently so it may rid itself of unhealthy fecal pockets (called diverticula) that often develop because of a sluggish condition.[5] Clearly, everyone would benefit in some way from taking alfalfa tablets (**caution:** do not use if you have problems with blood clots)!

Take four or five of them with every meal and crack them in your mouth before swallowing (if they are the type that can be). This will ease their digestion.

See the Recommended Vendor List to help you locate companies that carry high-quality alfalfa tablets; other brands also are available at most health food stores. Just buy them and use them! Your body will love you for it!

Nutrilite® is a registered trademark of Amway Corporation, Inc.

---

[3]Ibid., p. 72.

[4]Bernard Jensen, D.C., *Tissue Cleansing Through Bowel Management* (Escondido, California: by the author, 1980), p. 59.

[5]Bernard Jensen, D.C., *Doctor-Patient Handbook* (Escondido, California: Bernard Jensen Enterprises, 1976), p. 12.

CHAPTER 2

All Spices & Herbs (ASH)

Dr. Joseph Manthei, D.C., formulated this combination of more than 92 different herbs and spices that was intended for use as a condiment. It does not contain garlic or oregano because it was determined many people were allergic to them.[1] It is called All Spices & Herbs (ASH). You need to use it because it was designed to help the lungs.

The lungs need the greatest number of different minerals (84) to operate properly—more than any other organ in the body.[2] There is a wide variety of minerals present in the ASH seasoning.

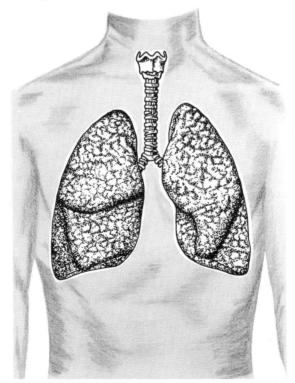

---

[1] Pamela S. Manthei, *Help From the Sanctuary* (USA: by the author, 1985), p. I-4.
[2] Dr. Joseph Manthei, *More Excellent Way Ministries: Home Correspondence Course* (Quarryville, Pennsylvania: by the author, 1978), p. 62.

Use this as a flavoring on your foods to boost the nutritional content. Sprinkle it on your salads or on your eggs. Add it to your soups or vegetables or casseroles as you prepare them.

This product is similar to blackstrap molasses (see Chapter 6) in that it is another easy way to add extra minerals to your family's diet.

CHAPTER 3

Aloe Vera

Aloe vera is often called the "healing" plant. Its sticky sap can be very soothing when applied directly to burns, cuts, or rashes of the skin. It also is useful when taken orally as either a juice or a gel.

The plant is light green in color, with long, slender leaves that are slightly serrated on the outside, and has a white spotting that runs its entire length. You can break a tip of the leaf off and apply it directly to your source of discomfort. Amazingly, the plant doesn't die, as it will "heal" the tear itself and continue growing. These hearty plants make a pleasant addition to any others that are decorating your household.

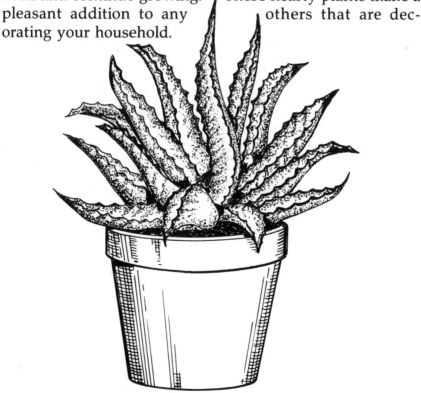

35 Practical Ways To Improve Your Health

The aloe vera contains allantoin, which is believed to be the basis of its healing power. The body uses allantoin to help increase cell growth. Comfrey tea (see Chapter 15) is another source.[1] Aloe vera contains magnesium, sodium, and potassium, which the colon needs to function properly (see Chapter 10)—also calcium, manganese, iron, zinc, and lecithin (see Chapter 34).

Almost anyone with digestive or elimination problems would benefit from drinking aloe vera gel or juice.[2] It has even been used to help shrink hemorrhoids.[3] Do not take any during the first three months of pregnancy, however, as its laxative action may induce an unwanted miscarriage.

Here is one way to drink it: Mix 1 tablespoon of aloe vera gel with 4 ounces of a carbonated beverage, such as 7-Up, Sprite, Canada Dry Collins Mixer, etc., and drink it twice a day between meals (it is believed that this method makes it easier for the body to absorb).[4] Or you can take 2 tablespoons a day of an aloe vera juice and mix it only with distilled water. Either method is fine.

Nature's Sunshine Products Aloe Vera Juice is one brand I like because 100% of the aloe gel is used to prepare it (check the Recommended Vendor List). You also can purchase a variety of other brand names at your local health food store.

While the aloe vera juice or gel is somewhat bland tasting, remember that it is a wonderful and easy way which nature has provided for you to improve your body's health internally and externally.

---

[1] *A Systems Guide to Natural Health* (Spanish Fork, Utah: Nature's Sunshine Products, Inc., 1988), p. 37.
[2] Carey A. Reams, with Cliff Dudley, *Choose Life or Death* (Harrison, Arkansas: New Leaf Press, Inc., 1978), p. 119.
[3] Ibid.
[4] Ibid.

CHAPTER 4

Bee Pollen

Being as busy as a bee is a cliche often used to describe someone who is very active. This, of course, is a favorable inference that the person has many industrious characteristics of one of nature's most important creatures: the honeybee.

The honeybee was given the responsibility for nature's pollination process, while moving from plant to plant, to be sure that these species would become fertilized and perpetuated. It does this service by inadvertently leaving behind male pollens from other plants and flowers that it has collected and stored in its back legs. This activity is essential to life on this planet as we know it.

After a hard day's work, the honeybee returns the pollen it has retrieved back to the beehive to store it for use as food. This also is where the beekeeper collects it.

Former President Ronald Reagan was the oldest person ever (at age 77) to hold the highest office in this country. He had a reputation for being in excellent shape and maintained a physical appearance of a man much younger than his years.

He suffered two major health traumas during his two terms in office. One occurred in 1981, when a bullet pierced his chest and partially collapsed a lung. The other involved a major colon operation he underwent in 1985. He recovered very quickly from both setbacks.

The nutrition product he has been taking since the early 1960s, and the one he attributes his good health and healing powers to, is none other than bee pollen![1] This is a good reason for you to consider eating it as well.

---

[1] Royden Brown, *How to Live the Millennium: The Bee Pollen Bible* (Phoenix, Arizona: Plains Corporation, 1989), pp. 117-119, 128-129.

35 Practical Ways To Improve Your Health

Bee pollen is called nature's perfect food. It contains all 22 amino acids including a high concentration of the eight essential ones (see Chapters 1, 14 & 25). It is plentiful in potassium, phosphorus, calcium, and magnesium and a host of trace minerals. It is one of the richest sources of the vitamins A to E, has essential fatty acids (see Chapters 14, 25, & 34), contains lecithin (see Chapter 34), and food digestive enzymes (see Chapter 11). It also is high in rutin (vitamin P). The body uses this to strengthen the walls of blood capillaries, which helps prevent strokes. One ounce of bee pollen contains about 90 calories.[2]

It is believed that bee pollen provides energy, helps slow down the aging process, rejuvenates the glands and skin, and leaves a person feeling relaxed and invigorated. It is a food that the whole body can use.[3]

Bacteria cannot exist in bee honey. The high potassium content kills the bacteria because it withdraws the vital moisture that they require for survival.[4] It also is an interesting fact that the honeybee will mix in a little honey with the pollen while collecting it.[5] This explains why bee pollen has long been renowned for being both antiseptic and sterile.

Mr. Reagan preferred one brand of bee pollen over all the others. It's called High Desert® Honeybee PollenS™ produced by the C C Pollen Company of Scottsdale, Arizona (see the Recommended Vendor List for their complete address).

The trademark on High Desert® Honeybee PollenS™ states that it is composed of "The Pollen of 10,000 Flowers!"® This pollen is collected from 20 different states to insure that the greatest variety of nutrient sources is obtained. It is processed very carefully to retain its vitality

---

[2]*Is Honeybee Pollen the World's Only Perfect Food?* (Phoenix, Arizona: C C Pollen Company, 1984), pp. 2-16.
[3]Ibid.
[4]D. C. Jarvis, M.D., *Folk Medicine* (New York: Fawcett Crest Books, 1958), pp. 99-100.
[5]*Is Honeybee Pollen the World's Only Perfect Food?*, p. 2.

and keeps well (you can even freeze it for long-term storage). It is sweet and easy to use.

Warning: Do not use bee pollen if you have ever had an allergic reaction or suspect any sensitivity to it. The company recommends the following guidelines to use if you're not sure:

> Take just 1 granule for 7 days. Double it during the next 7 days, and continue doubling it for the next several weeks. After doing this for 2 months, your daily intake would be about 1 teaspoonful or 1/6th ounce (3 teaspoons to a tablespoon, 2 tablespoons to an ounce). You can gradually increase the amount you use based on how you are feeling.

Use about 1-2 teaspoons a day. The pollen granules are available in either one or five pound packages. You also might want to try "The President's Lunch™ Bar" (it was named for Ronald Reagan), which is a nutritious and delicious diet snack containing bee pollen.

Whichever of their fine products you choose (they have a variety), find a way to include bee pollen as a part of your regular diet. You should notice an improvement in your health by using it.

CHAPTER 5

Belief In Someone Higher Than You

You are a product of your creation. By that I mean you are the sum result of your thoughts, attitudes, and belief systems. Therefore, I feel that any discussion about improving the quality of your health has to include the raising of your spiritual awareness. This means believing in Someone higher than you.

Have you ever taken a good look at the world you live in? Have you ever noticed the blue color of the sky, watched clouds lazily float by, or experienced the freshness of the air you are breathing? Can you remember the carefree sounds of children laughing and playing, which could only bring a smile of contentment to you as well? These are all expressions, in our lives, of the Supreme Being that I have chosen to call the God force. I use this term because I believe it is a more representative definition of His energy and presence. The western world's version is far too limited and restrictive.

The God force reveals himself to us daily, on this beautiful planet, if only we could recognize and learn to appreciate this fact. Everything that we see, smell, hear, and feel was created in His perfection for our enjoyment! Anything less than beautiful or perfect, is a result of something that humankind has produced.

The Creator created us to enjoy perfect health also! Yet the general health of the people in this country is not as it should be. Perhaps that is one reason you are reading this book.

35 Practical Ways To Improve Your Health

If you've ever had the opportunity to spend time studying the human body or the powerful effect that nutrition has on it, then you know how humbled you can feel! The body is the most complex, yet perfect organism on the face of this earth! In Psalms 139:14, David says simply: "For I am fearfully and wonderfully made." So too, is the rest of us!

The body's stamina is truly amazing. It can be nutritionally mistreated, and even starved for years, yet miraculously recover when fed the right foods. A good example is those people who suffered in concentration camps during World War II, yet somehow recovered. If not for our bodies' instinctive will and resilient spirit to survive, gifted to us through the loving grace of the God force, how else could this be?

It's time for the people in this country to return to the basics of health. I'm referring now to our spiritual health, as well as nutritional. We need to recognize that good health is not a right, but a blessing given to us by our merciful Maker. If we choose to continue to break or ignore His laws of living in harmony with nature and each other, then they will continue to break us.

You need to consider the relationship between you and Him if you are serious about improving your health. Ask for guidance and discipline as you make changes in your diet. He will listen and he will help! I firmly believe you won't dramatically change your health level until you do!

CHAPTER 6

Blackstrap Molasses

Blackstrap molasses is a by-product of the juice of sugar cane, after the majority of any granulated sugar has been separated from it. Thus, it contains all the nutrients and about 70 trace minerals that have been removed from the more commonly known white sugar product.

It is very high in iron and potassium, and is an inexpensive way to add these important minerals to your diet. If you are drinking raw goat's milk, be sure to include the blackstrap molasses with it to replace the iron that is missing (see Chapter 24).

Try taking it straight or mixed in a cup of hot water. It does taste different, but it doesn't take very long to get used to. Dr. Carey Reams had a favorite saying about those times when a person was trying to decide if they would eat a new food or not: "Teach your tongue who's boss!"

To those words of wisdom I would add: "You are not eating or drinking certain foods because they taste good; you are eating or drinking them because they are good for you. And there is a difference." I taught my tongue who is boss and I have a tablespoon in the morning.

Use the blackstrap molasses as a condiment to increase the nutrition content of the food you are cooking. Store it in a squeeze bottle near your stove and add it whenever you like. Don't put it in foods that will look unappealing with it, such as grits or cauliflower. Still, you can include it in the water of other vegetables or foods you are preparing, as appropriate. Be careful not to use too much as it can overpower the flavor of the food you are mixing it with.[1]

---

[1] Pamela S. Manthei, *Help From the Sanctuary* (USA: by the author, 1985), p. I-3.

35 Practical Ways To Improve Your Health

I use Plantation Blackstrap Molasses that you can find at most nutrition stores. Some grocery stores are carrying it now also. Do not buy the brand of molasses that contains sulphur. This is because the sulphur could be good or bad for you depending on your body chemistry type.

CHAPTER 7

Cayenne Pepper

In the herbal world, cayenne pepper is referred to as capsicum. It is known as red pepper. Whatever it's called, it is a wonderful stimulant for producing energy in the body.

Cayenne is beneficial when used to help stop any unnatural internal or external bleeding that may be occurring in the body. It also is well known to have a positive effect on a person's heart and blood pressure, as it opens circulatory passages in the body, especially the upper portion. In fact, cayenne has been used successfully to increase circulation to ulcers of the stomach, which then helps them to heal.

Dr. A. B. Howard, author of *Herbal Extracts*, writes of the famous study that was done about the use of cayenne: "The renowned doctor and surgeon, William Beaumont, observed in his now classic observations of the stomach through a hole which formed after a gunshot wound to a young fur trader that Cayenne does not irritate in any way the lining of the human stomach despite its sensation of great heat.... Increased circulation to the stomach gives it a healthy pink glow, not to be mistaken for irritation."[1]

How ironic that the very food that is often shunned by those with stomach or digestive problems, because of its reputation for being too hot, is the very substance that the body may need to help repair itself!

Capsicum is identified as the purest and best stimulant among all herbs, according to author Louise Tenney in her book *Today's Herbal Health*.[2] In *Herbally Yours*, by Penny C. Royal, she says it can act as a catalyst, with other herbs, to help the body use them all better.[3]

---

[1] (Berkley, Michigan: The Blue Goose Press, 1983), p. 32.
[2] 2nd ed. (Provo, Utah: Woodland Books, 1983), p. 38.
[3] 3rd ed. (Provo, Utah: Sound Nutrition, 1982), pp. 20-21.

35 Practical Ways To Improve Your Health

Cayenne contains the following nutrients: potassium, iron, calcium, magnesium, phosphorus, sulphur, vitamins A, B-complex, and C.

Use the cayenne as a condiment that you can add to your casseroles or soups or whatever, for flavoring. You also can purchase the capsicum as an herb and take it as a daily supplement. Look at the Recommended Vendor List to find who can supply it. Or you can check with your local health food store to see what they carry. Always buy it organically grown.

Use the cayenne pepper where and when you can. It is a very simple but wise addition to your diet.

CHAPTER 8

Change Your Attitude

This is easy to say, but often difficult to do. Still, I consider this concept so important that I have decided to identify it as a key area that must be addressed before you can make any real progress toward improving your health.

What effect on health does one's attitude have? Every day we make choices about the ultimate direction our lives will take. These choices influence the attitude we develop toward certain areas of our existence. Therefore, it is our attitude that can and does decide whether we choose to live a healthy or an unhealthy lifestyle, and I think it's important to realize that.

If you are serious about feeling better again, then it is going to be essential that you begin to change your attitude about the whole issue of what is good health.

A person has to work really hard to become sick. That's right! You have to work consciously at breaking most every natural law that your Creator set in motion, which if followed, would have provided you a life filled with vitality and good health.

These laws cover every aspect of life: spiritual, physical, nutritional, mental, love, emotional, energy, and balance. They bring peace and happiness to the body. However, because they are the God force's laws, they also can break a person's health if one chooses to continue to ignore or violate them. And you need to be aware of that.

Though they can't be seen, or touched, or smelled, they exist as surely as the minuscule molecules that make up the very paper that you are reading these words on. The chapters in this book will identify ways for you to become in harmony with these laws again.

35 Practical Ways To Improve Your Health

Dr. Bernard Jensen often uses the following expression when referring to a person's outlook on life: "Your attitude is your altitude." So, your attitude dictates your level of consciousness, in all matters including your health. At what level would you currently place your health?

You need to consider changing your attitude about the way you view different aspects of health—primarily the foods you now eat, and sometimes, of even more importance, the foods that you don't!

You most assuredly are going to have to change your previous eating habits because this is what got you into trouble in the first place. You are going to need to be more open-minded about what is or is not good for your body and then make changes in your diet that reflect this new awareness.

This will not be an easy task to accomplish. Still, I have always believed that whenever something is too easy, it's probably not worth pursuing anyway. It may be reassuring for you to know that real change usually takes place as a process anyway, and not as an event.

Now this doesn't mean that you will have to change your whole lifestyle overnight, only that you must be willing to keep an open mind about different ideas that you may have no experience with. And you won't be required to give up all your previous beliefs either, just resolve to approach new ideas and information, without judgement, until you can decide how they will fit into your new health understanding. First you must open your mind, then you can change your attitude! This is the key.

Accept the fact that you may have been wrong in your previous ideas about nutrition, and then move on. It is OK to admit that you were wrong. I believe it is not so important to know from where you are coming; rather, it is *more* important to know where you are going. No one has all the answers all the time, and to think one does is an unrealistic and unhealthy way to view the world.

Change Your Attitude

Change can cause discomfort, that cannot be denied. It involves the rethinking and redoing of ordinary tasks. You may become discouraged trying to incorporate these different changes into your new health lifestyle, but remember this: You had to learn how to crawl before you could walk, and how to walk before you could run. For now, do what you can when you can, and let it go at that.

I believe there is a correlation between learning how to change one's attitude and one's ability to receive and understand wisdom and knowledge. Dr. Jensen has an interesting observation on this subject: "Wisdom is the ability to discover an alternative." Still, alternatives are only discovered after a person has become open-minded enough to change their attitude!

As you review the following pages, use your new "wisdom" as the basis to consider changing some of your previous habits. This is your first step to a healthier lifestyle.

I have always tried to live my life using a very simple idea: If you notice something about yourself that you don't like—change it! Just like that—just that simple! The choice is yours. And only you can make that choice.

I believe you can change your attitude; now it's time for you to take that responsibility, believe it yourself, and **MAKE IT HAPPEN!**

CHAPTER 9

Chlorophyll

Chlorophyll is the material that gives a plant its green color. The basis for all life begins during photosynthesis, or the interaction of sunlight with chlorophyll, which in turn manufactures food energy for the plant.

Chlorophyll is an excellent blood and circulatory system builder as well as purifier. It contains vitamin A, E, K and magnesium that is strikingly similar to the same makeup of human blood except that it contains iron. Yet, this difference does not prevent it from being converted into blood, because a switch of the magnesium and iron molecules will take place.[1] It also is a rich source of several nutrients including potassium.

For anemic conditions, a complete blood builder can be prepared by mixing liquid chlorophyll with a little black cherry juice (it is very high in iron). This combination also is good for the nerves.

Animals have a very highly developed sense of smell. There is a belief that fear generated in a frightened animal generates an acid that can be sensed by other animals stalking them. Chlorophyll acts as a natural deodorizer in the body. Dr. Bernard Jensen tells one story that substantiates chlorophyll's unique masking qualities: "There is chlorophyll on a new born baby deer. This coats and screens the fear acid so it will not be killed prematurely by predators."[2] Therefore, the chlorophyll protects the baby deer until it is strong enough to flee its pursuers on its own.

It is believed that chlorophyll has a positive effect on the pancreas by helping it to regulate and control the sugar level

---

[1] Dr. Bernard Jensen, 80th Birthday Symposium, San Diego, CA, 08-27 to 09-01, 1988.
[2] Ibid.

in the body. It helps relieve pain too.[3]

The list goes on about the varied benefits of this wonderful tonic that nature has provided for us. Make it a part of your daily health regimen.

Most of the retail liquid chlorophyll products come from organically grown alfalfa (see Chapter 1). I have a liquid teaspoon in a glass of distilled water every morning.

---

[3] Dr. Joseph Manthei, *More Excellent Way Ministries: Home Correspondence Course* (Quarryville, Pennsylvania: by the author, 1978), p. 81.

CHAPTER 10

Cleanse Your Colon

The colon, or large intestine, has long been the "butt" of many a snide comment or bad joke (oops, looks like I just did it too!). Perhaps its negative connotation goes back to the early childhood "toilet training" we all received or how Society, in general, has always regarded it. Whatever, one way or another, many of us were left with the impression that the lower bowel in our body was something "bad" or "dirty." It clearly was not something that you would ever seriously discuss with another person.

There is an interesting characteristic that is common to the liver, lungs, kidneys, heart, spleen, etc., and the colon as well: they are all considered as organs of the body. Plain and simple, the large intestine is an organ in your body in the same way that your heart is. It has its own unique functions to do and was created perfectly by your Creator as he created all the other parts of your body.

The colon is responsible for the removal of harmful toxins and undigested food materials from the body. Its normal functioning is essential for keeping the body's health in complete harmony. You would become very ill if it was unable to do this. Here then is a brief description of the various segments that comprise the colon (see next page).[1]

The small intestine is responsible for most of the digestion of the nutrients needed by the body. It winds its way through the lower body cavity until the ileum, or final section of the small intestine, joins with the large intestine in an area known as the cecum. This connection point on the lower right side contains, appropriately, the ileo-cecal valve that opens and closes to regulate the release of any

---

[1] Bernard Jensen, D.C., *Tissue Cleansing Through Bowel Management* (Escondido, California: by the author, 1980), pp. 12-18.

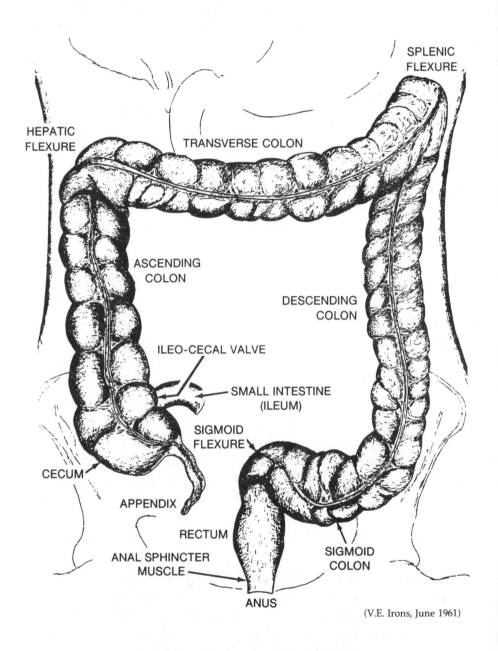

(V.E. Irons, June 1961)

A HEALTHY COLON

Cleanse Your Colon

undigested foods into the colon. The appendix is nearby and has two important functions. It acts as an "oil can" that lubricates the ileo-cecal valve[2] and also produces and emits a germicidal fluid that neutralizes any toxic food material entering the cecum.[3]

The ascending colon begins from here moving straight up toward its first turn to the left. This is identified as the hepatic flexure (which means "turn") because it changes direction very close to where the liver is located.

It then moves from right to left across the body cavity, at a slightly elevated angle, and is called the transverse colon. It makes another turn downward on the left side of the body at what is termed the splenic flexure. This is because the change takes place near the spleen.

The descending colon now moves toward the lower bowel area and crosses back over to the right where it positions itself in about the middle of the body. This occurs at a slightly lower location than where the cecum on the other side of the body is situated. This is the sigmoid colon area, and is known as the "holding tank" because wastes are stored here until it is time to release them.

The colon moves downward again, changing direction at the sigmoid flexure. The rectum continues from this point, in the shape of an "S," until it becomes the anus that is the rectal waste opening. The anal sphincter muscle is present here that opens and closes the anus. From end to end, the large intestine measures about 5 feet long with a diameter of about 2 1/2 inches.

Dr. Bernard Jensen, besides other doctors, believes that a malfunctioning of this elaborate elimination system is responsible for many current maladies and illnesses that afflict us.[4] He feels a proper functioning colon is the key to improving a person's health, and often suggests changes in

---

[2]Bernard Jensen, D.C., Ph.D., *Your Personal Neuro-Optic Analysis*, "The Cecum."
[3]Norman W. Walker, D.Sc., Ph.D., *Colon Health: The Key to a Vibrant Life* (Prescott, Arizona: Norwalk Press, 1979), pp. 88-89.
[4]Jensen, D.C., *Tissue Cleansing Through Bowel Management*, p. 1.

his patients' diets and lifestyles that would help rejuvenate the colon. He considers it one of the most neglected organs in the body.[5]

I have known several people who have told me that they have a bowel movement (BM) every third day, or even every sixth or seventh day and that this is normal or OK for them. I would answer that by saying if their colon is healthy and operating in the manner for which it was truly intended, they should be having a minimum of one to three BM's a day, and it would be even better if they had one after every meal they ate!

It does not make any sense nor appear logical to hold waste materials in your body for a week and then to assume that this will not have a negative effect on you. A constipated colon is a primary cause of diverticulitis (see next page), and could even result in a complete blockage of the colon. It can even induce a diarrhea that the body will manifest in an attempt to cleanse itself.[6]

Diverticulum (singular) or diverticula (plural) are pencil-like protrusions of impacted fecal material that have pushed through the actual wall of the colon. This abnormal bulge would look similar to someone's index finger sticking straight out, after it had been poked through the inside of a rubber inner-tube (see drawing). Diverticulosis of the colon means that diverticula are present.

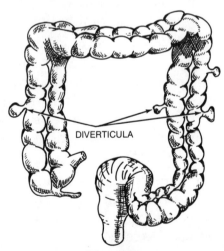

Diverticula
By permission of Dr. Bernard Jensen, D.C., Ph.D.,
(From *Tissue Cleansing Through Bowel Management*)

---

[5]Bernard Jensen, *Nature Has a Remedy* (Escondido, California: by the author, 1978), p. 67.
[6]Robert Gray, *The Colon Health Handbook*, 6th ed. (Oakland, California: Rockridge Publishing Company, 1982), p. 8.

The diverticula often become inflamed because of the fecal matter that gets trapped in them.[7] This infectious condition is named diverticulitis and has been recognized as the cause of many complications throughout the body. If the fecal matter is kept moving through the large intestine, with BM's that are regular and complete, you will not have this problem. Alfalfa tablets are one of the finest foods to aid in the elimination of diverticula (see Chapter 1).

They do this by providing the much-needed fiber or bulk, and nutritional support, that is necessary to strengthen the walls of the colon to the point where they can expel any fecal impactions. The fiber forces the muscles of the bowel to squeeze and contract harder—in effect, creating an exercise program for the colon that works from the inside-out. The colon needs three major mineral types to function optimally: magnesium, sodium, and potassium. They are all represented in the alfalfa with many other vital and trace minerals.

A sluggish bowel also can contribute to allergy problems. When the colon is ignored, the level of toxins in the blood starts to rise because they are not being eliminated. Consequently, they begin backing up into the skin and lymphatic system, which are not capable of handling such an overload, and this often produces an unfavorable reaction (see Chapter 29).

It is now necessary to stress the importance of eating a properly balanced diet that has raw, whole, and pure foods (see Chapter 25). Be sure to eat more salads (see Chapter 23) or foods that add roughage to your diet. The fiber from raw vegetables and fruits will act as a broom to help "sweep" out any waste materials that may be attaching themselves to the walls of the large intestine. They also contain gelatin that will act as a natural lubricant or oil for the stool. This results in easier eliminations, and is one reason that salads should be eaten first before the regular meal.

---

[7]Jensen, D.C., *Tissue Cleansing Through Bowel Management*, p. 37.

35 Practical Ways To Improve Your Health

There is a reason for everything that happens in the body. If the colon is constipated, then eating the right foods will help get it moving again. Foods which are yellow in color, such as bananas, squash or beans are slightly laxative.[8]

Have a warm glass of prune juice or even steamed prunes to start your day. Avoid high sugar, processed or unnatural foods as they slow down your elimination system. Use bread sparingly, as it coats the lining of the intestine and interferes with its normal rhythm.

Cascara Sagrada is an herb that is used to stimulate peristalsis action, which is the involuntary movement of the contents within the bowel. It does this naturally by strengthening the sphincter muscle. Use it cautiously—it has a powerful cleansing action on the body. It is easy to take in its capsule form. Start with a small amount and increase gradually.

There is an excellent tea that can be very soothing and helpful to an irritated colon. It is called flaxseed tea (see Chapter 14 on how to prepare it). It is wonderful for cases of diarrhea, gas, or anything else that may be bothering your digestive or elimination system. Flaxseed is high in silicon, calcium, potassium, and vitamin F (omega 3 & omega 6) that is very effective in healing the tissues of the intestinal tract. The seed also contains a slippery substance useful for softening the stool.

The entire body, with all its different organs, must work together and in harmony. Dr. Jensen contends that when one organ is underactive, it produces a strain on all the others.[9] This means that a weakened organ can actually produce a negative "reflex" type of action in another part of the body.[10]

There is a belief by some, including myself, that one of the various causes of the severe headaches that people

---

[8]Dr. Bernard Jensen, *Creating a Magic Kitchen* (Escondido, California: Bernard Jensen Enterprises, 1973), p. 17.

[9]Dr. Bernard Jensen, 80th Birthday Symposium, San Diego, CA, 08-27 to 09-01, 1988.

[10]Ibid.

suffer through is directly tied to problems starting from an underfunctioning bowel. Many people, after completing colon cleansing programs, have happily reported that their long-standing migraine headaches disappeared after their bowel problems were corrected. Some would call this cause and effect.

The colon cleansing program these people used is very simple. It usually involved the taking of a plant fiber, such as psyllium hulls (or husks), with plenty of water. The water causes the psyllium to swell and expand, and as it moves through the large intestine it scrapes and dislodges mucus and other hardened fecal matter that have stagnated there. You would not feel anything unusual while this is happening.

Typically, some type of cream or herb is used in conjunction to help loosen this material from the walls of the bowel. Many systems include the use of a clay, called bentonite, which is very effective in absorbing toxic materials.

A form of friendly bacteria, known as lactobacteria or acidophilus, also is taken because it too, is removed by the psyllium but is necessary to ensure the well-being of the intestinal tract. The acidophilus is needed to control the putrefactive bacteria, known as coliform, which can cause bowel gas.

If you suffer from this condition, it means that your colon needs attention and that you are lacking acidophilus.[11] Use it whenever in your diet, even if you're not cleansing. I take some every day.

I believe everyone could benefit from a cleanse of their colon because it can help correct constipation or diarrhea problems. The American diet of fast, fiber deficient, devitalized food has contributed to the poor condition of this elimination system. If you suffer from allergies, cleansing your colon may bring the relief you seek.

---

[11] Gray, pp. 17-19.

There are many fine cleansing programs that you could use and they will not interfere with your daily routine. I have completed one as explained in the book *The Colon Health Handbook,* by Robert Gray.

Nature's Sunshine Products has a pre-packaged ten-day cleanse that is simple-to-follow and gentle on your system. I highly recommend it for first-time cleansers who are either skeptical, or feel uncomfortable about the whole process.

Dr. Jensen uses a formula that has been very effective. Most health food stores will have some type available (the cleanse should contain only natural ingredients). Look around and compare. Be sure to check with your doctor before starting.

You need to consider doing this! The chapter on "Change Your Attitude" has prepared you. Be willing to be different, think different, and do different. Take care of your colon; its proper functioning is essential for you to maintain a high level of health.

CHAPTER 11

Digestive Aids

Digestive aids provide essential food enzymes, a dilute hydrochloric acid (HCl), or protein "splitters" that the body needs to digest and absorb its food properly. Enzymes exist naturally in all foods that are in their raw state. Yet, because so many foods eaten in this country are processed, or cooked, there is a deficiency of these important enzymes in most people.

A good enzyme supplement would include several or all the types listed below that are necessary to break foods down to their corresponding nutrient level:

protease enzymes ...... proteins
amylase enzymes .... carbohydrates
lipase enzymes .... fats
cellulase .... fiber

(or any variation of these four types)

They work best when taken with the meals. Use two capsules, tablets, or powdered servings when the food is eaten raw, and four when it is cooked.

The HCl is stored in sacs in the lining of the stomach. A sufficient amount must be available to lower the acid pH level of the stomach, and activate an enzyme found here called pepsin. Pepsin is important because it digests proteins. Once again, however, a person's diet, with the stresses of modern day living, affects the quantity and quality of the acid that is available. It is believed that about 80% of people over the age of 45 have a deficiency of HCl.[1]

Some manufacturers include pepsin with the HCl, some do not. Either way, it is recommended that you take the HCl about 15 to 45 minutes after you finish your meal depending on the individual. This ensures that the digestive process is correctly prepared to receive it.

---

[1]Dr. Bernard Jensen, Basic Iridology Seminar, Toronto, Ontario, 06-23 to 06-25, 1989.

Another excellent digestive aid to use is papaya (preferably green and unripened). It contains all the digestive enzymes, plus a protein digestive enzyme known as papain. Papain's digestion of protein is superior to pepsin because it occurs in any type of stomach environment: acid, alkaline, or neutral. It does not depend on the body's production of HCl.

During the digestion process, the papain converts some of the protein into an amino acid named arginine. An ample supply of arginine is necessary to stimulate the pituitary gland to produce the human growth hormone (HGH). HGH is essential in the regeneration of RNA, DNA, and liver, muscle, and cartilage tissue. Exercise (Chapter 13) enhances its ability to increase muscle mass, as it reduces body fat.

If you were to eat an ideal variety of raw, whole, and pure foods (see Chapter 25), it's conceivable that your diet would not be deficient in the enzymes or protein digestants. Still, regardless of your present eating habits, just about everyone could benefit by taking these digestive aids.

Incidentally, it is better for you not to drink water or liquid of any kind while eating your meals, as this can result in an upset stomach, indigestion, or gas. The extra moisture dilutes the stomach's digestive juices, and prevents the parotid glands from producing enough saliva that is necessary to help predigest the food. Instead, drink the water between the meals; you should notice a difference in your digestion almost immediately.

Enzymes International, Inc., of Manitowish Waters, Wisconsin, and Nature's Sunshine Products carry very good food enzyme, HCl, and papaya digestive aids. They are available in either tablet, capsule, or powder form, depending on the company (see the Recommended Vendor List).

Eating the right foods is the first step to increasing your health level. Yet, it's just as important that these foods are digested properly. I highly recommend using digestive aids to help you reach your goal of a healthier body.

CHAPTER 12

Distilled Water

We have been provided with a multitude of blessings in this country. Natural resources, vast food reserves, and an abundance of pure, clean water. As with all things, however, when something is taken for granted, there is a risk of forever losing it. Such has been the case with this nation's drinking water.

It is encouraging that this country has finally begun to realize the importance of cleaning up its water supply. Yet, it has been contaminated and polluted to such an extent that all water sources are now suspect, and you need to be aware of that.

Years ago, my mother told stories to me of how she and her mother would collect rain water from barrels around the side of their house and use it to wash their hair. She remembered how soft and refreshing it felt. The water they collected was rain that fell from clouds that was completing the natural distillation process that occurs every day around the world.

The water was basically pollution free—not only to wash hair in, but to drink as well. Unfortunately, she probably wouldn't feel safe doing that today because of the air pollution particles that the rain now merges with as it falls to the earth.

Questions also are being raised about the current municipal water supplies that are being "treated" with chemicals that are supposed to protect you from tooth decay, bacteria and other human-made pollutants. This is akin to treating a disease with another disease.

The water molecule is very powerful. For example, anything that it contacts, such as a pollutant or contaminant, is trapped within and held tightly. It is, therefore, very difficult to force the water molecule to release that impurity.[1] Distillation is the only water treatment that fully does this.

Here's why: Water is heated in a boiling chamber to 212 degrees Fahrenheit. Steam slowly rises and passes through a coil that wends its way about a circulating fan. The cool air causes the higher temperature water vapor to condense where it is collected and stored below in a container. Through this process, the water molecule is forced to separate itself from anything that has a higher or lower boiling temperature, and leaves behind the contaminant.

The principle used in producing distilled water is patterned after nature's hydrological cycle. Water evaporates from the surface of the oceans or lakes and rises above to the atmosphere. The water vapor is formed into clouds until it condenses again as rain moisture and returns to the earth to repeat the cycle. Distillation, then, is nature's way of purifying water for this planet.[2]

There are other types of bottled water available on the market today. For example, spring water is very popular. It is often stated that it is a good source of minerals for your body. Still, I question which minerals are present in the water, and in what proportion? I believe the God force put foods on this earth to provide us with the minerals we need to sustain life, and not the water.

While it's true that the spring water may contain some natural minerals, it may be as true that unnatural materials, such as toxins or antigens, also are present. The problem is, you can't really be sure.

The liver has to purify everything that you eat or drink. One of its major functions is to ensure that any toxins are filtered and removed from the blood. This means it also would have to process anything that is contained in the water, such as a natural mineral that can be used later

---

[1] Eldon C. Muehling, *Water for the Eighties: A Cause for Concern* (Lincoln, Nebraska: Kane Associates, 1979), pp. 1-3.
[2] Esther Dougherty, *You Have a Right to Know*, rev. ed. (Lincoln, Nebraska: Kane Associates, 1980), p. 29.

Distilled Water

somewhere in the body, or an unnatural toxin that has to be disposed of through one of the elimination channels. Whatever it is, of course, will require the liver to work and expend energy.

One immediate advantage to drinking distilled water is that it requires very little effort or energy by the liver to cleanse it, since the water has already been purified. Now this doesn't mean that it is 100% pure, only that it is very close to this figure. Therefore, taking distilled water will help preserve your energy for use in other areas.

Distilled water benefits the body in other ways also. You are composed of two-thirds water, roughly equivalent to the same amount that covers this earth. Pure water is essential to the metabolic process that occurs in your body to produce a new cell.[3] It acts as a "catalyst" for the correct amino acid combinations to form that are necessary to replace your worn-out and damaged cells.[4]

This fact should finally put to rest, completely, the often stated argument used against distilled water that implies it will "leach out" vital minerals from within the cells. This is nonsense! In fact, the purer the water is, the easier it will be for the body to rebuild itself, produce healthier cells, and then remove the old ones.[5]

Most people don't drink enough water. A good guideline to follow is to take your weight and divide it by two. Change that number to ounces and drink that much water every day. For example, if you weigh 160 pounds, you should be drinking 80 ounces consumed evenly throughout the day (4 ounces every half hour). Drink no more than this amount even if you weigh more. Any vegetable or fruit juices, including other liquids you drink during the day, would count toward this total; just make sure that at least

---

[3]Carey A. Reams, with Cliff Dudley, *Choose Life or Death* (Harrison, Arkansas: New Leaf Press, Inc., 1978), p. 42.
[4]Reams, p. 46.
[5]Dr. Allen E. Banik, *The Choice Is Clear* (Kansas City, Missouri: Acres U.S.A., 1975), p. 32.

half the ounces come from distilled water. If you have a tendency toward low blood carbohydrate, then drink less or add natural sweeteners such as honey or maple syrup.

By increasing the amount of water in your diet, you also will stimulate your kidneys to release any troublesome toxins and acids that have collected in the body (drinking a little diluted cranberry juice helps too). Do not be alarmed if you find yourself making more trips to the bathroom. This is a natural response from the body. One of the reasons people get a kidney infection is simply because they are not drinking enough water.

Some people complain that they don't like the taste of distilled water. If you think about it, pure water is colorless, odorless, and tasteless. What they are tasting is nothing more than bacteria or loose material in the mouth that is being washed over their taste buds. This usually lasts for only a couple of days.

The distilled water is sold in plastic containers. There also are stainless steel water distillers that allow you to produce it in the privacy of your home. See the Recommended Vendor List for a price comparison between the two.

Your goal is to improve your general health condition. You realize the importance of eating foods that are as pure as possible (see Chapter 25). It only makes sense that you also should be drinking the purest water that is obtainable for your body. And that means distilled water—period!

CHAPTER 13

Exercise

It would be wise to consider the role that regular exercise plays in a healthy lifestyle. Perhaps you have a real aversion to any type of strenuous, physical exercise. I'm not going to raise your anxiety level by insisting that you join the local aerobics club. I am going to suggest that you try something else that can be as beneficial for you, if not more so.

One of the finest total exercises you can do is walk! That's it!! Period! This is my great revelation!

A vigorous half-hour walk everyday will do more for you than you might believe possible. Your legs are known as the "pumps" of the body. That is, they contain the largest muscles in the body and were designed to help circulate the blood throughout your system. When the blood is circulated, it is forced into the brain area that is the most difficult area for the heart to reach because of something known as gravity.

It is believed that a major reason people get ill is that they are not getting enough blood to their head.[1] Walking helps and encourages this action.

Former President Dwight Eisenhower's doctor had this to say about the human body: "Show me a person with flabby leg muscles, and I will show you a person with a flabby brain."[2] He understood the importance of regular exercise as well.

You may say that you are too tired to do even your daily activities, let alone consider walking for thirty minutes a day. This is a prevalent attitude of many people who do not exercise. Still, there is a certain amount of irony associated with this point of view, because I believe the way to get

---

[1] Dr. Bernard Jensen, 80th Birthday Symposium, San Diego, CA, 8-27 to 9-01, 1988.
[2] Ibid.

energy is to expend it!

That's correct! The more you exercise, the more energy you will have!!! It almost sounds too good to be true! The energy is generated as a direct result of the action of the body being in motion, which increases the demand for more blood. This, in turn, raises its oxygen content, and produces a feeling of well-being. It is as simple as that!

So the more you walk, the better you will feel. One reason you may be tired is that you're *not exercising!* Think about that for a moment...

Prove it to yourself! Check with your doctor first, then set a moderate goal to begin walking. It may be for only one block, or for only ten minutes. It doesn't matter, just start.

Be sure to invest some time and money in a good pair of walking shoes. A cheap pair of foot apparel will do more harm to a beginner's exercise program than anything else.

This does not mean buying an inexpensive pair at your neighborhood discount store; go to a shop that specializes in athletic footwear. This assures you of proper fitting shoes. Start your exercise program, correctly, from the feet up! You'll never regret it.

Develop a definite time and day that you do your walking. You will get better results if you set a regular walking schedule and then follow it (see Chapter 27).

Walk with your spouse, loved ones, friends or even your pet. If you walk by yourself, buy a low-priced radio headphone or cassette and play your favorite music. This is very relaxing.

Start slowly and gradually build your distance and duration. Set a goal of at least 30 minutes a day and then decide for yourself if you are feeling better. I believe that if you follow a consistent walking schedule, you will notice a dramatic improvement in your general attitude and health!

CHAPTER 14

Flaxseed

One of the finest foods that you can use for your gastrointestinal tract is flaxseed. The seeds are small, brown, oval shaped, and they are prepared as a tea, or added as a supplement with other foods. They contain a high amount of silicon, potassium, and calcium. They also have vitamin F (unsaturated and essential fatty acids) that is useful for healing the tissue of the intestines. Flaxseed is mildly laxative.

Because of the rich silicon make-up, you will notice that the seeds are very shiny. This means the flaxseed is helpful for your skin, hair, nails, glands, and nervous system that all require this important mineral. My mother remembers using the flaxseed as a wave set for her hair. A favorable characteristic of the flaxseed tea is that it is very soothing. Is it because of its high silicon content?

The real beauty of the flaxseed is the way it is used to help regulate both diarrhea and constipation conditions. It really is the God force's gift for any lower bowel elimination problems.

The tea is very useful to control diarrhea. This is how you make it:

> Add 2 tablespoons of flaxseed to a pint (2 cups) of boiling distilled water.
>
> Reduce heat and let simmer for about 7-10 minutes.
>
> Strain the seeds from the tea and throw them away.
>
> The tea will be somewhat thick and bland tasting.
>
> Store remainder in refrigerator; drink it cold if you desire.

35 Practical Ways To Improve Your Health

Here is another approach to making the tea. Add a quarter cup of flaxseed to a one quart container filled with hot water and then let it stand overnight. Again, the seeds are strained and thrown away. This method preserves the fullest amount of the Vitamin F.[1]

The flaxseed can be used for relieving ordinary constipation too. The seed will swell to about three times its original size when it is mixed with water or other liquids and will provide desirable bulk for the colon to work with. It also produces a jelly-like substance that helps to lubricate the stool for an easier elimination.

It makes a fine addition as a supplement that can be sprinkled on your hot breakfast cereals or salads. Add one or two teaspoons as desired. It may be run through a grinding mill if you have access to one.

There are approximately 50 essential nutrients that the human body needs to survive. They must come from the foods we eat, because the body cannot make them by itself. Two of them are identified as essential fatty acids (see Chapters 4, 25, & 34). The linoleic acid form, known as omega 6, is very plentiful in our diets. Raw sesame seed butter (see Chapter 31) is a good source for it.

The linolenic acid, or omega 3, is often scarce. According to Dr. Paul Stitt, founder and owner of Natural Ovens of Manitowoc, Wisconsin, flaxseed is very high in omega 3 and contains some omega 6. He uses whole ground flaxseed in several of his natural breads and other products. Write or call him from the Recommended Vendor List at the back of this book, to see if his goods are available in your area.

You may remember hearing before about omega 3. It recently gained national recognition when derivatives of it (EPA and DHA) were identified as very prevalent in the traditional Eskimo diet. These derivatives are found at high levels in the cold water fish that they are so fond of.[2]

---

[1] Bernard Jensen, *Nature Has a Remedy* (Escondido, California: by the author, 1978), p. 73.
[2] Paul Stitt, M.S., *The Power of Flax*.

Flaxseed

There is a belief that omega 3 plays an important part in reducing heart attacks and strokes by helping prevent blood platelets from sticking together when they are not supposed to. It is interesting that heart problems are almost unheard of with the Eskimo, although their diets contain much fat.[3]

The body requires eight essential amino acids too. Flaxseed is an excellent source of these vital nutrients (see Chapters 1, 4, & 25).[4]

Flaxseed can deplete the body of vitamin B-6, and the metabolism of omega 3 requires zinc of which it contains very little. Be sure to include extra of both as a supplement to your regular diet.

If you prefer, flaxseed also is available as an oil. Always buy it cold-pressed, and keep the flax oil sealed and refrigerated since it is susceptible to becoming rancid. Cold-pressed is an extraction process that uses minimal heat to help guarantee that the nutritional value of the oil is not destroyed.

You can find flaxseed in most health food stores or co-ops, but read labels carefully before purchasing. Obtain only the finest, organically grown flaxseed available. It is worth every penny you spend because you will be providing something very nutritious and helpful for your body.

---

[3] Ibid.
[4] Udo Erasmus, *Fats and Oils* (Vancouver, British Columbia: Alive Books, 1986), p. 264.

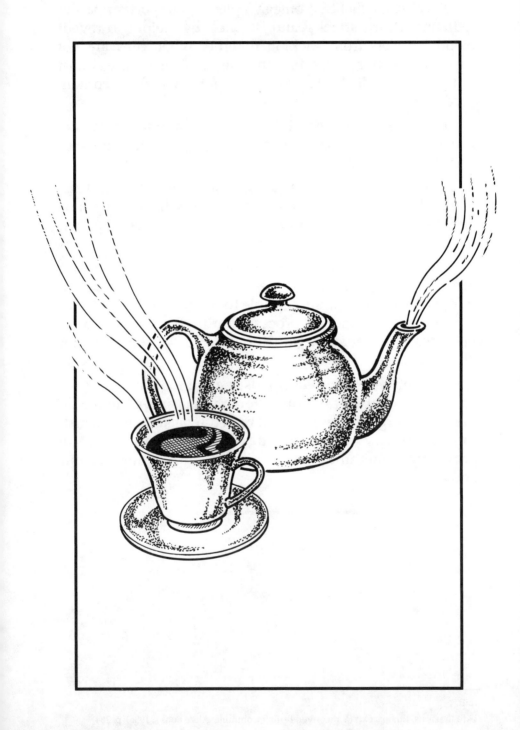

CHAPTER 15

Herbal Teas

The following herbal teas can be used as a refreshment with your regular diet. They may be sipped throughout the day, whenever you like, and are a good way to increase your body fluids. They also provide nutritional support to many different bodily systems.

There are a variety of ways to make your tea (follow the printed instructions if you buy it prepackaged). Here is just one of many:

> Fill your stainless steel or glass teapot with hot water (this heats it up separately). In addition, use a kettle to boil freshly drawn distilled water.
>
> Empty the teapot and put in 1 or 2 good-sized teaspoons of your favorite tea.
>
> Add 1 or 2 cups (depending on how strong you like it) of the water from the kettle the moment it boils; this ensures that the water will be hot, yet still loaded with enough oxygen to extract the full flavor and benefit from the tea. Never directly boil the herb.
>
> Let this steep for about 5 to 10 minutes (longer if indicated), stir and drink it warm or cool (store it in the refrigerator), whichever you prefer.
>
> Include a little raw honey or lemon if you wish to flavor it.

Some teas, such as flaxseed (see Chapter 14), will require the use of a stainless steel strainer after brewing. For others, use the strainer to hold the tea as you pour the hot water through it. A tea ball strainer or tea infuser spoon works well also.

35 Practical Way To Improve Your Health

Here then, is a list of those teas that I believe are the best of the best, and the parts of the body that will benefit:

Oat Straw Tea (Avena sativa): hair, skin, glands, nervous system, nails

Have you ever noticed the sheen of a horse's coat as it glistens in the sunshine? It is a beautiful sight. Did you ever consider what is a major food that a horse is fed? The answer is oats!

Oats are very high in silicon and this is what gives the horse's hair its shininess and vitality. Look at a field of ripening oats sometime; you'll notice that it also glistens in the sun. This is the same silicon you see only now it is coating the outside of the oat straw stem.

You can have hair that lustrous too. This tea can help you get that, as it is one of the richest sources of silicon available.

Flaxseed Tea: stomach, large and small intestine, nervous system

This tea has already been discussed in detail (see above reference).

Hawthorn Berry Tea: heart, circulatory system

This red berry has been renowned for years as a heart strengthener. It may be somewhat difficult to locate as a loose tea, still it is often available in a capsule form that can then be made into a tea.

Peppermint Tea: oxygenator, digestive system, nervous system[1]

It has a very pleasant, refreshing taste.

Comfrey Tea: general healer in the body

Comfrey has long been revered for its broken bone and wound "knitting" capabilities. It is high in calcium and is one of the finest teas to drink.[2] Do not use this if you have a

---

[1] Penny C. Royal, *Herbally Yours*, 3rd ed. (Provo, Utah: Sound Nutrition, 1982), p. 37.
[2] Louise Tenney, *Today's Herbal Health*, 2nd ed. (Provo, Utah: Woodland Books, 1983), pp. 48-49.

tendency toward low blood carbohydrate, as it may lower it even further.[3]

Dandelion Tea: liver, gall bladder, blood purifier

Yes, this is made from the leaves and roots of those yellow weeds that grow wild in your backyard! It works as a detoxifier in the body.

Alfalfa Tea: digestive system, elimination system, balanced nutrition

Chapter 1 discussed the merits of alfalfa in detail.

Pau D'Arco Tea: immune system

Indigenous to South America, it also is known as Taheebo tea. It is very high in iron.

Horsetail (Shavegrass) and Uva Ursi Tea: kidneys, bladder

It would be better if you refrained from drinking the commercial iced tea products and other teas such as the orange pekoe or black. They are very hard on your kidneys because of the tannic acid that they contain. Tannic acid causes the cells in your kidneys to swell and reduces the flow of urine. Chocolate contains it too, along with a caffeine-like substance called theobromine.

Why not take something that would help the kidneys instead? These two teas have been used as diuretics and cleansers for the body. The horsetail has a high silicon content.

Cornsilk Tea: kidney, bladder

It is helpful for dissolving stones found in these important eliminative organs.

Red Raspberry Tea: pregnancy, female organs

This tea is useful for strengthening the uterus and for relieving other ailments associated with pregnancies. It is slightly diuretic and considered beneficial to those women who have difficult menstruations.[4]

---

[3]Dr. Joseph Manthei, *More Excellent Way Ministries: Home Correspondence Course* (Quarryville, Pennsylvania: by the author, 1978), p. 69.
[4]Tenney, p. 106.

The taste of these teas will vary from bland to refreshing. Remember, just because something tastes sweet doesn't mean that it is good for you. Refined sugar is a perfect example.

Learn to eat and drink foods that will make you healthier and forget what they taste like. You will be surprised at how quickly your taste buds will adjust when you learn to stop resisting changes to your diet.

You can purchase these bulk teas at most health food co-op stores. Bring a container. Many of these varieties also are now available as gelatin capsules that will dissolve in the tea water (use from 2-4). Nature's Sunshine Products is an excellent source. Again, buy the finest organically grown that you can and expect to pay for it. If it's not available, then use what is.

The above teas will vary in price depending on the variety, but they are all worth it. Remember, a little will last you a long time.

It's OK if I didn't mention your favorite tea. Everyone has their preference. What is important is that you drink several different teas. The greater the variety, the better chance your body will receive the right nutrients it needs from the teas.

The true value of any herbal tea is in how it provides you with easy to use nutrition while supporting weakened body systems. Try as many as you can! You won't regret it. They are a viable and positive way to enhance your health improvement program.

CHAPTER 16

Iodine

The thyroid gland needs an adequate supply of iodine for it to operate correctly. Whenever there is a shortage, the thyroid cannot properly use the hormone thyroxine that is essential in the regulation of the body's metabolic system. This system controls the speed of your bodily functions.

Accordingly, if there is an iodine deficiency in your body, there is probably a thyroxine imbalance as well. This may result in a person who is always tired with a very low energy level. They may have problems in staying warm since it is very difficult for their body to generate any heat. They could have a weight problem too.

Thyroid problems also can be the cause of dry, lifeless hair or affect the menstrual cycle of some women. It is very important to consider the condition of your thyroid if you are serious about raising your health level.

The thyroid regulates calcium in the body, and whether it is hypoactive (underactive) or hyperactive (overactive) always requires iodine.[1] If it is hypoactive, it lacks iodine; if it is hyperactive, it is consuming a high amount of iodine and will need more. Anyone over the age of 45 should be sure to include more iodine in their diet.[2]

The oceans contain a rich source of this water soluble mineral and sea kelp (brown seaweed) is one of the best ways to get iodine. It is an abundant source of a variety of minerals and vitamins. You can buy it at most health food stores. When used as a condiment, it makes an excellent salt substitute.

Carrots grown in California have a higher parts per million (ppm) content of iodine than those grown in any

---

[1] Dr. Bernard Jensen, Basic Iridology Seminar, Escondido, CA, 10-28 to 11-01, 1988.
[2] Dr. Bernard Jensen, 80th Birthday Symposium, San Diego, CA, 08-27 to 09-01, 1988.

other part of the country. The soil there is very rich in iodine because of its proximity to the ocean. This is another easy way to increase the amount of iodine in your food.

Dr. Bernard Jensen uses a purple colored seaweed, known as dulse, in his iodine supplements that also is high in manganese. It is available in either a powder, liquid, or tablet form and in many different sizes. Whichever product you decide to purchase, use it as a regular addition to your daily diet.

CHAPTER 17

Learn To Love

The desire to be loved by others is one of the most basic needs of people. It implies acceptance and substantiation of each of us as individuals. It also implies that we must love others in return. I believe that you will never reach your full health potential until you understand and practice this very basic principle.

To love others, you must first learn how to love yourself. Now I am not referring to a narcissistic form of love that is directed only at yourself, but one that realistically identifies and accepts your weaknesses and also your strengths. This means learning to like and accept yourself as you are.

You can accomplish this change by removing the negative thought patterns that you may have allowed to become ingrained in your subconscious mind. Start by seeing yourself as a beautiful person, one who can love and be loved; for what you think you are is what you will become!

By learning to love others, you will find it easier to eliminate these negative thought patterns. Dr. Bernard Jensen has this to say about why it is so important to remove them: "Every thought you think will find a point in your body." He knows that any destructive or negative thought that you allow into your daily life will ultimately find a place in your body and cause an adverse side effect.

How can this be? I believe it is because we are beings of energy. This means everything we do or think is an expression of energy! And if the thoughts we think can become a form of energy, then they can help or interfere with the proper functioning of the body depending on whether they are of a positive or negative nature.

Dr. Carey Reams understood this principle when he described it this way: "Hatred is the finest seed that cancer ever had!" So, if you are the type of negative individual who holds grudges, or cannot forgive others when they make mistakes, or even harbors hatred toward your fellow brother or sister, then you run the terrible risk of destroying yourself from within! Cancer could be the result of the negative thoughts and energy that your body is creating!

I believe that loving others sets in motion the natural Law of Love that is the most powerful force governing this planet. It provides for the giver to receive as much or more love than they gave and ensures that their emotional needs will be met. It confirms the oft quoted biblical scripture: "It is more blessed to give than to receive."[1]

Cynics would ridicule this by saying there is no proof of any such law since nothing can be seen or felt or heard because of it, yet others would answer that they have been "touched" by the love of other people, or "felt" the presence of love, or have even been "in love" themselves. So something doesn't always have to be "real" before it is believable.

Dr. Jensen relates a story of an interesting lesson that his mother taught him about loving others. After asking him what he had learned that night after returning from a church gathering, he told her: "I learned to love my friends and love my relatives and love my enemies...." She said, "Son, sit down; I want to talk to you. I want to tell you that you do not have to love everybody." "Oh, mother," I said, "that doesn't sound very good." She said, "You know, you don't need to love your friends, relatives, or your enemies, son; you need to love for your own good."[2] So, don't love others just for their sake; learn to love them because of the good it can do for you also.

---

[1] *Holy Bible: King James Version* (Cleveland, Ohio: The World Publishing Company), Acts 20:35.
[2] Bernard Jensen, D.C., Ph. D., *Master Feeding Program* (Escondido, California: by the author, 1988), p. 6.

Learn To Love

Learning to love is essential for your emotional, physical, spiritual, and mental well-being. To love and be loved is to experience those magical and wonderful feelings that are an inherent right of every human being. It is the ultimate gift that was given to us by the God force. In most ways, it *represents* what the God force really is! And what could be more perfect than that?

Perhaps you have some personal relationships in your life today that are not right. Remember the price in health that you and the other person are paying for these disagreements. Make a resolution to resolve these differences this very minute! Because you love yourself and because you need to love others...

CHAPTER 18

Liquid Minerals

Your body needs minerals to function correctly. They are nature's building blocks that provide nourishment and support for the body at the lowest cellular level. There are several ways to be sure that you are receiving an adequate supply. Eating a variety of foods would be a good place to start, but sometimes, because of time constraints within our daily schedules, this is not always possible.

There is a better and more reliable way to support your regular diet with the correct minerals your body requires. It is by ingesting what are known as liquid minerals.

Liquid minerals represent exactly what their name implies. They are a liquid mixture that contains a variety of essential minerals, including many trace. They are very concentrated and usually not very pleasant tasting. Their tastes can be masked, sometimes, by mixing them with other liquids such as a juice, but don't depend on it. The best time to take them is after your meals.

An advantage of this form of mineralization is that they are made available to the body in a very short period provided they are in a natural, easily digestible form. The body does not have to expend much energy to use them.

There are several reasons for this. If you have ever browsed through a health food store, you may have noticed that many supplement products say they are chelated. Chelation means the molecules of these minerals are bonded in a complex structure with carbon to make it easier for the body to assimilate them.

Bonding occurs when an electron from a molecule with a lower specific gravity or "atomic weight," overlaps and links with electrons in the field of a molecule that has a

35 Practical Ways To Improve Your Health

higher specific gravity (such as iron or manganese). This is important because the lower the specific gravity of a mineral, the smaller the molecule and the better the body can extract it. The chelated mineral acts like a train engine that "drags" the heavier and larger sized mineral (caboose) behind it, thus enhancing its digestion. Chelate comes from the Greek word "chele" that means "claw."

You may have seen minerals identified as colloidal also. A colloid, when referenced as a type of measurement, is an extremely small particle. Consequently, minerals in a colloidal form are very easy for the body to process and use because of their minute size (see Chapter 19).

You must be careful not to take too many liquid minerals, however, as they can start a diarrhea in the body because the quantity is too intense for it to handle. If this happens, either the body is trying to exchange toxic materials for the new minerals, very rapidly, or it has become overwhelmed and will do everything it can to eliminate these also. Whatever the reason, just cut back on the quantity you are taking until it is under control again.

Mostly, they will make a fine addition to your daily mineral intake from other foods. It is important that you take food enzymes (see Chapter 11) with the liquid minerals, at least one tablet, capsule, or powdered serving per ounce. This aids in their digestion. I drink mine in the morning.

There are two different products on the market that I am familiar with and use (see Recommended Vendor List). Enzymes International, Inc., produces an excellent liquid mineral (both chelated and colloidal). Their product is derived from mineral deposits found in an ancient seabed.

Another good one is Marine Minerals. Theirs is produced from minerals found in the Great Salt Lake of Utah. It is interesting that a person's blood contains almost the identical minerals as found in salt water. In fact, during World War II, there were instances when seawater was used as a replacement for blood plasma, and the patients lived.

Liquid Minerals

Marine Minerals are much more concentrated than the Enzymes International, Inc., and have had 99.5% of the sodium removed. Their minerals are in an ionic (very small and non-chelated) form, but also are high in electrolytes such as magnesium. Electrolytes are essential for your body because they conduct and maintain electrical energy that your cells need to stay healthy. I drink a mixture of the Marine Minerals and distilled water, after running or exercising, to help restore my electrolyte balance.

Despite which one you choose, they will both provide additional mineral support whenever you need it. A stable source will always be necessary if you wish to see any significant improvement in your total health.

35 Practical Ways To Improve Your Health

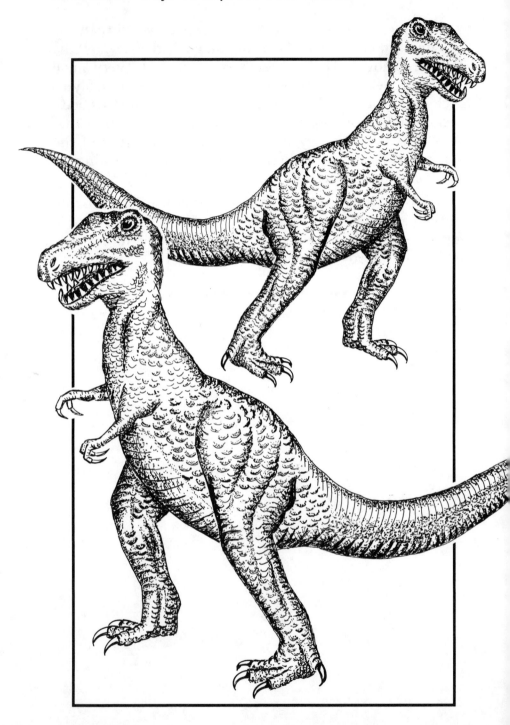

CHAPTER 19

Min-Col

Dr. Carey Reams recognized the importance of minerals in a person's diet. He was determined to discover a source that would provide a balanced formula that worked in harmony with the body, and he did. It is called Min-Col.

Min-Col is actually the essence of bone meal. If you had a ton of bone meal, that essence would equal about 60 pounds. Manufacturers can only retrieve about 3-4 pounds of Min-Col from that small amount.[1]

There are 66 different minerals present in Min-Col—all in a phosphate form that is easily accepted by the body. This is because their biochemical structure is very compatible with the body's chemistry and requires little change.

Several of them, specifically phosphate of calcium and phosphate of fluorine, are essential for strong bones and teeth.[2] If your fingernails break or tear easily, or have white spots on them, then this is an indication that you could use Min-Col.[3]

The minerals are provided in what is known as a colloidal form (see Chapter 18). They are so small that they are similar to the dust that our Maker created us from.[4]

It is interesting that the soft rock phosphate that contains this colloidal material was present in another form many years ago. It is the remains of dinosaurs which once roamed this planet![5]

The origin of these fearsome dinosaurs, and especially

---

[1] Carey A. Reams, with Cliff Dudley, *Choose Life or Death* (Harrison, Arkansas: New Leaf Press, Inc., 1978), p. 117.

[2] Dr. Joseph Manthei, *More Excellent Way Ministries: Home Correspondence Course* (Quarryville, Pennsylvania: by the author, 1978), pp. 73-74.

[3] Manthei, p. 74.

[4] Joseph C. Manthei, D.C., *Health Through Diet* (Quarryville, Pennsylvania: More Excellent Way Ministries, 1983), p. 18.

[5] Manthei, *More Excellent Way Ministries: Home Correspondence Course*, pp. 74-75.

35 Practical Ways To Improve Your Health

their sudden destruction about 65 million years ago, has puzzled scientists for many years. Their bones supplied the raw material that was necessary for the current development of Min-Col. This is my explanation of how and why it all occurred. You won't find this story in any school geology book.

Genesis, Chapter 1, verse 1 of the King James Version of the Bible states: "In the beginning God created the heaven and the earth." Verse 2 continues: "And the earth was without form, and void; and darkness was upon the face of the deep."

These two verses appear to be in conflict, because I Corinthians 14:33 says: "For God is not the author of confusion." God is the father of harmony and not the disharmony that verse two suggests the earth had fallen into. If God was not responsible for the conditions as explained in this biblical passage, who was? We know it wasn't Adam and Eve, the first man and woman, because they were not created until verse 27.

Part of the answer is tied to a belief that verses 1 & 2 speak of a great difference in time. Verse 1 tells of God's initial creation of the earth and the universe. Job 38:4, 7, say that His angels ("sons of God") shouted for joy during this event, which means they existed long before man was ever created. Verse 2 refers to a much later date when the earth is in disarray.[6]

The English translated word of "was," as recorded in Genesis 1:2, is from the Hebrew word "hayah." Yet, when "hayah" was used in other places throughout the Bible, it was given a correct translation of "became" to show something had changed. Biblical scholars are now recognizing the difference and have retranslated this important verse to read: "Now the earth **had become** waste

---

[6]Robert E. Gentet, *Dinosaurs Before Adam?* (Pasadena, California: Ambassador College, 1972), pp. 6-7.

and empty."⁷ This new interpretation clearly shows that a dramatic change had somehow occurred to the earth after its original perfect creation.

Isaiah 14:12-14 discuss the rebellion that the high angel Lucifer (later to become Satan) and his other angels waged against God to overthrow him. Verse 13 talks of Lucifer's specific attempt to ascend to heaven and exalt his *present* throne "above the stars [angels -Ed.] of God." This plainly says that he was already in a position of authority (over the earth) during this time in question.⁸ He was, of course, defeated and verse 12 explains the fate that befell him and the angels who followed him: "How art thou fallen from heaven, O Lucifer,... how art thou cut down [back -Ed.] to the ground [earth -Ed.],...!"

The second half of verse 2, Genesis, Chapter 1, describes how God begins again the recreation of the earth and the subsequent removal of the chaos (i.e., when the dinosaurs reigned over this world) that Lucifer had allowed. It begins with: "And the Spirit of God moved upon the face of the waters." The rest of Chapter 1 details God's establishment of a new order, which included man in the image of himself.

I believe this is the explanation for what caused the worldwide mass extinction of the dinosaurs and ultimately led to the formation of the soft rock phosphate that is now called Min-Col. How ironical, yet perfect, that our Father would create a beneficial mineral supply from the ashes of prehistoric animals that were never part of his Divine Creation.

Most present-day bone meal supplements are derived from cow bones. They often contain traces of lead, and other toxic materials, because the cows lived and ate foods produced in a world contaminated by agricultural

---

⁷Herbert W. Armstrong, *Did God Create a Devil?* (Pasadena, California: Worldwide Church of God, 1978), pp. 2-3.

⁸Herbert W. Armstrong, *Mystery of the Ages* (Pasadena, California: Worldwide Church of God, 1985), p. 67.

chemicals, automobile exhausts, and noxious, smoke-belching factories. Lead, like many other hazardous by-products, has a natural affinity for bones.

The bone meal found in Min-Col is of a purer extract, as it is obtained from creatures that flourished in a time and environment that was pollution free. This is another good reason to use it.

Min-Col can be given to children or adults. Here are the suggested guidelines to follow, depending on the age of the person:[9]

> For babies 2 months and up, until they can take it orally, open the capsules and rub it on the soles of their feet (the largest pores in the body are in the feet and the colloidal mineral can be absorbed right through them).
>
> Children from 6 months to 4 years can use 1/2 capsule/day until the child is 4 and then 1 capsule/day until puberty, which the boy can continue with, but the girl should increase to two/day for the rest of her life.
>
> Children between 4 and 10 can take two/day for three to four weeks, and then one/day until puberty, which the boy can continue with, but the girl should increase to two/day for the rest of her life.
>
> For ages 10 to 40, use 2 capsules twice/day for 60 to 90 days, then two/day for the rest of their life.
>
> For adults over 40, take 2 capsules twice/day for anywhere from three to six months and then two/day for the rest of their life.
>
> As a reminder: If you are pregnant, double your intake to 2 capsules twice/day. This will ensure a sufficient supply for both mother and child.

---

[9]Manthei, p. 74.

Do not be concerned about taking too much of the Min-Col as it is non-toxic and whatever is not used is passed out through the bowels. You can order the Min-Col directly from Dr. Joseph Manthei. Check the Recommended Vendor List for his full address.

This planet has been blessed with a very wonderful mineral supplement: Min-Col. It has given me a greater appreciation and understanding of Genesis 2:7 that states: "And the Lord God formed man of the dust [colloidal? -Ed.] of the ground, and breathed into his nostrils the breath of life;...." To continue your healthy existence, consider including Min-Col as a part of your day-to-day nutrition.

CHAPTER 20

Niacin Flush

It is acknowledged that niacin (vitamin B-3) produces a flushing effect that drives blood to all parts of the body. One only needs to see or feel the flush that is easily evident after it is taken, especially on an empty stomach, to know this is true.

This increase in circulation will provide only benefits for the brain and extremities, which are difficult areas for the heart to reach, and the internal organs. The increase in the blood supply carries vital nutrients that are necessary to support these systems properly.

The niacin causes a dilation (opening) of the blood vessels and capillaries that, of course, are essential to an adequate blood source throughout the body. It forces the blood to move into the most minute areas of the body and carries away any impurities it finds.

Do not take the niacin on an empty stomach. This will usually help minimize the effects of a flush to the head. When one does occur, it normally lasts only a short time (about 30 minutes). You need to start gradually on this program so any flushing will not cause undue discomfort.

Some people also have complained about an itching sensation that occurs during the flush (as the vessels begin to dilate). If this happens, use a natural bristled skin brush (see Chapter 29) and give yourself a good brushing. This will help.

Use the purest form you can get as many brands contain unnatural fillers. And don't buy the time-release. You want the benefit of an immediate flush, not a slower version. The brand I use is NatureMost® Laboratories Inc.

If 100 mg. is the smallest tablet that you can get, and you need 50 mg., just cut it in half.

35 Practical Ways To Improve Your Health

NOTE: Check with your physician before starting this program:

1) Take a 50 mg. tablet with the breakfast meal and another 50 mg. with the supper (total 100 mg./day). Have it 3/4 of the way through a meal or after the meal. Use a full glass of water and do this for 3 days.

2) For the next 3 days take 50 mg. with the breakfast, lunch and supper meals (total 150 mg./day).

3) For another 3 days change to 100 mg. with the morning meal, and 50 mg. at the noon and evening meal (total 200 mg./day).

4) Now increase to 100 mg. for all three mealtimes during the next 3 days (total 300 mg./day).

5) If you are not having any problems with these proportions, then you may continue to increase it gradually to a maximum of 1000 mg. (or 1 gram) a day provided it does not cause you extreme distress.

6) Any noticeable flushing to the head should diminish within 3 or 4 days. If the flush does not go away, then allow more time before you increase the amount or just use what you can stand until your body adjusts.

CHAPTER 21

Onion Soup

Most of us are aware of the important role that vitamin C plays in keeping us healthy. We have been taught that a cold is an indication of a vitamin C deficiency, and I believe that, but this is only one of the signs.

Vitamin C has been called the collagen or "glue" that holds your body cells together. When there is a vitamin C deficiency, the ears may droop, the lips will become thicker, the tongue develops a coating on it, or there are stretch marks in the skin. These are external signs of an inward vitamin C deficiency.[1]

It has been determined that the richest source of vitamin C is contained in an onion. It is even more highly concentrated than in acerola cherries, citrus fruit, green peppers, or rose hips![2]

This is an onion soup recipe that is used for extracting as much of the vitamin C as possible:[3]

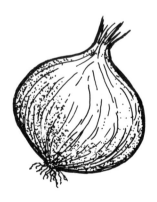

To 3 cups of distilled water, add 4-5 medium size, organically grown, chopped onions.

Simmer for 15-20 minutes until the onions are soft and transparent.

Add either some fresh or frozen vegetables, herbs (such as basil or parsley), a small amount of broth

---

[1] Dr. Joseph Manthei, *More Excellent Way Ministries: Home Correspondence Course* (Quarryville, Pennsylvania: by the author, 1978), pp. 76-77.

[2] Manthei, p. 77.

[3] Dr. Joseph Manthei, *More Excellent Way Ministries: Diet Booklet* (Quarryville, Pennsylvania: by the author, 1978), p. 16.

> powder (e.g., Dr. Bernard Jensen's Broth or Seasoning) and then a small amount of margarine for flavoring purposes.
>
> Combine other nutritious foods or condiments such as barley, eggplant, whole-grains, blackstrap molasses (see Chapter 6), or ASH (see Chapter 2) as desired.

Despite your body chemistry type, this soup will nourish it with the necessary vitamin C. It is a simple, yet very effective way to be sure that you or your family's vitamin C requirements are being met. Consider it another piece of the key that can open your door to a happier and healthier lifestyle.

CHAPTER 22

Potato Peeling Broth

Potato peeling broth is very high in potassium and silicon. Potassium is known as the "great alkalizer." It is very effective in helping the kidneys drain the body of acids that have accumulated, unlike another mineral, natural sodium, which helps to neutralize them.[1]

It is highly recommended to use the broth during times of a fever, or for those who suffer from extreme arthritis or rheumatism. The heart, because it is a muscle, requires potassium too and benefits as well.[2]

Sixty percent of the potassium in a potato is directly beneath the surface. When potatoes are peeled, much of the potassium is lost. By using the skins of the potato, you are getting the highest potassium broth possible.[3]

Potassium is bitter, so expect it to taste different.

Here is the recipe:[4]

This broth can be taken between meals, right with your regular diet, and should be made fresh daily:

> Use 3 large, organically grown, red potatoes (never make broth with green potatoes).
>
> Slice peeling 1/4" thick (throw the center of the potato away; this is the acid part).
>
> Use 4 carrots, 8 sticks of celery and a handful of parsley.

---

[1] Bernard Jensen, Ph. D., *The Chemistry of Man* (Escondido, California: by the author, 1983), p. 327.
[2] Ibid., p. 294.
[3] Ibid., p. 295.
[4] Ibid., p. 294.

Place all of this in about a quart and a half of distilled water.

Bring above to a full boil, lower the temperature and simmer for 20 minutes.

Strain liquid off and drink about one pint daily for 30 days.

CHAPTER 23

Rainbow-Colored Salads

A rainbow-colored salad contains exactly what its name implies. It would include a full complement of vegetables with colors that match those of the rainbow. They would be raw, whole, & pure as possible (see Chapter 25).

Here is a sample of those vegetables with their naturally occurring colors:

>orange - carrots, squash
>green - celery, leafy lettuces, spinach, broccoli, sprouts, cabbages, chard, cucumbers, beans, peas, peppers, etc.
>yellow - wax beans, squash, peppers
>red & purple - tomatoes, peppers, radishes, cabbage, beets, onions
>white - cauliflower, radishes, onions

By combining these color variations in one salad, you will guarantee yourself a balanced vitamin and mineral meal because nature uses color to express its nutritional structure.

Vegetables that are orange and yellow in color are high in vitamin A and considered laxative. Vegetables which are red and green will help to rebuild the blood. If they have seeds, such as cucumbers, green beans and peas, or squash, then they contain manganese. Foods that are black, like raisins or olives, have iron in them. Be sure to include some of these in your salads also.

All vegetables provide a good variety of necessary nutrients. When you combine them, your body is assured of receiving the full benefit of a nourishing meal.

It is better to use only leafy lettuce (red leaf, romaine, bib, etc.) instead of the more common iceberg head. The leafy lettuce contains 100 times more iron and 80 times more chlorophyll than the head lettuce. The head lettuce has very little nourishment, slows down the digestion process, and causes gas.[1]

The next time you prepare a salad, plan ahead when you buy the vegetables to be sure that a variety of colors is represented. This is an easy and fun way to increase the aesthetic quality of what you are eating while improving its nutritional content.

---

[1] Bernard Jensen, D.C., *A New Lifestyle for Health & Happiness* (Escondido, California: by the author, 1980), pp. 70, 98.

CHAPTER 24

Raw Goat's Milk

Many of us were introduced to cow's milk when we were just babies. Every school child was taught that milk is very high in calcium and is necessary for good health.

As adults, we are becoming more aware of the drawbacks to drinking milk. Many babies, myself included, have suffered through the unpleasant experience of an allergic reaction to milk (see Chapter 35). It can cause allergies in grown-ups too.

Cow's milk also produces mucus. It has even been thought that the negative aspects of drinking milk might outweigh the positive; yet, what would the alternative be?

Why not drink raw goat's milk instead? It is presently consumed by more than two-thirds of the world's population, yet most people in this country are not even aware of it.

Visualize for a moment the characteristics of a cow... Did you think of a large, heavy, plodding, slow-moving animal? Dr. Bernard Jensen says they appear that way because they are a *calcium* animal. Calcium is used in the body to make it hard and rigid, like your bones and teeth.

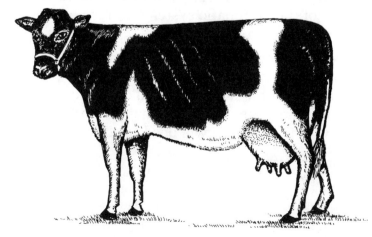

35 Practical Ways To Improve Your Health

Now, clear your mind again and think of the characteristics of a goat. Did you get an image of a limber, energetic, playful, fast-moving animal? Dr. Jensen says goats are *sodium* animals. Sodium is used in the body to keep it soft and pliable, like your joints. Notice a pattern here?

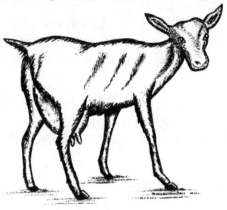

That's right! Raw goat's milk can help to keep your bone joints limber and supple because it has the highest amount of usable sodium of any food. I'm talking about natural sodium now, not sodium chloride or table salt! This is one of the reasons why Dr. Jensen recommends drinking goat's milk to so many of his patients.

The stomach requires sodium and if sufficient quantities of it are not available, it is unable to secrete enough hydrochloric acid (HCl) that is necessary to digest proteins properly (see Chapter 11).[1] Sodium also is the major ingredient of the lymphatic system[2] and is needed to keep calcium in solution for the body.[3]

There are other reasons to drink goat's milk other than for its sodium content. If you have a child that is allergic to cow's milk, try some raw goat's milk instead. Its chemical makeup is almost identical with that of mother's milk (all milk is low in iron, so you will need to add some blackstrap

---

[1]Dr. Bernard Jensen, 80th Birthday Symposium, San Diego, CA, 08-27 to 09-01, 1988.
[2]Dr. Bernard Jensen, Basic Iridology Seminar, Toronto, Ontario, 06-23 to 06-25, 1989.
[3]Bernard Jensen, Ph. D., *The Chemistry of Man* (Escondido, California: by the author, 1983), p. 343.

Raw Goat's Milk

molasses, Chapter 6, to raise the level). It produces little mucus, and there are very few babies who cannot tolerate it.

Fluorine is an essential mineral that is necessary for our teeth, bones, and immune systems. It is found in cow's milk, but leaves very quickly when heat is applied to it. Raw goat's milk contains 10 to 100 times more fluorine than cow's milk, and this is one reason it is best to drink the milk in its natural, raw state.[4]

Phosphorus is a requirement for the brain and nervous system, but is very difficult to locate in vegetables. It must come from a more highly evolved organism, such as an animal.[5] Goat's milk is abundant in it. It is highly recommended for those people on a vegetarian diet.

The fat globule of the goat's milk is only 1/6 the size of fat globules found in cow's milk.[6] Dr. Jensen says the milk also is very high in calcium, which is the mineral your body needs more of by weight and volume than any other. He likes it because it has all the necessary nutrients to "feed the whole body."

The sooner you drink it after it is milked, the better it will be for you. Dr. Jensen has stated that he's "seen the dead raised" with warm, freshly drawn goat's milk. Yet, he feels that it starts to lose some of its nutritional properties only 20 minutes after it is milked, so try to get it as fresh as you can.[7] If necessary, you can even freeze the goat's milk without sacrificing all the qualities of it.

There aren't any good reasons not to drink the milk, other than sometimes it can be difficult to locate a supplier. If you cannot find one, use a product known as Whex® because it is an excellent substitution. Whex® contains goat whey, which is the clear liquid that remains after cheese or cottage cheese is made. It is one of the highest sources of

---

[4]Dr. Bernard Jensen, Basic Iridology Seminar, Toronto, Ontario, 06-23 to 06-25, 1989.
[5]Jensen, Ph.D., *The Chemistry of Man*, p. 273.
[6]Dr. Bernard Jensen, Basic Iridology Seminar, Escondido, CA, 10-28 to 11-01, 1988.
[7]Bernard Jensen, *Nature Has a Remedy* (Escondido, California: by the author, 1978), p. 144.

sodium and potassium. The whey is dehydrated and you mix it with hot water for a nutritious drink (see the Recommended Vendor List to obtain it).

Some people will complain that goat's milk has a different taste to it than cow's milk. This is to be expected. As with all foods, your taste buds will adjust and you won't even notice the difference.

There is a belief that drinking raw unpasteurized milk could be dangerous because of any harmful bacteria or virus it might contain. Most goat milk producers have to follow a very strict schedule of testing for their goat herds, so the chances of this happening are very small.

I buy the milk from a local producer who lives on a farm away from the city. Minnesota does not permit the sale of raw goat's milk in a store (it does allow pasteurized), but there are states, such as California, which do. You may have to do some investigating to find a supplier, as Minnesota also restricts them from advertising except by word of mouth. A good place to start is your local health food store or co-op.

Goats, and their milk by-products, have a long, rich history. Deuteronomy 31:20 and Joshua 5:6 affirm the Lord's convenant to Moses and Joshua that he will lead the children of Israel into the promised land of (raw goat's) milk and (unheated) honey (see Chapter 4). That incentive, of renewed health and vitality through raw goat's milk, is still available for you today.

CHAPTER 25

Raw, Whole, & Pure

It is very important that most of the food you put into your body be as raw, whole, & pure as possible. Observing this rule is essential if you expect to improve your general health condition.

Whenever possible, eat your food in its natural, raw, uncooked form, unless your digestive system cannot handle this. Some people do better on a diet that includes cooked food, especially if they are sick or old. Prepare your foods in the way that is right for you.

Raw foods are important because they contain essential food enzymes (see Chapter 11) that are destroyed whenever heat over approximately 116 degrees is applied. The nutrients found in food will not be digested or utilized correctly unless these food enzymes are present.

If you choose to include cooked foods in your diet, consider these three common sense guidelines when making them:[1]

1) always use low heat
2) use very little water
3) use stainless steel cookware, with a lid when cooking, to retain the nutrients

Prepare the food whole because this is the way nature provided it and this also is the way it was designed to be eaten. The processing of whole wheat flour, brown rice, and sugar cane, to produce whitened, nutrient deficient products, is a good example of why the whole food should always be eaten.

---

[1]Bernard Jensen, Ph.D., *The Chemistry of Man* (Escondido, California: by the author, 1983), p. 192.

35 Practical Ways To Improve Your Health

One of the most nutritious foods you can eat is an egg yolk. It feeds the whole body and it contains the eight essential amino acids that are usually lacking in the diets of vegetarians (see Chapters 1, 4, & 14).[2] It is the richest source of phosphorus,[3] which also is present in raw goat's milk (see Chapter 24), and contains the essential fatty acids (see Chapters 4, 14, & 34).

What about the cholesterol we hear so much about today that is present in eggs? While it is true that eggs have a high cholesterol count, it also is true that right next to it in the yolk is some of the highest amount of lecithin (see Chapter 34) found in any food, which will break this down.[4] So nature has produced a balanced, nutritious food for us, provided we eat it correctly.

Because high heat is the enemy of lecithin, the way in which you prepare the yolk is very important. Eat them poached or soft boiled, so you won't destroy the lecithin and the other valuable nutrients. Do not fry the egg because then what you have is the cholesterol without the lecithin.[5] Lecithin received its name from the Greek word for egg yolk.[6]

Commercial egg factories produce eggs that contain more cholesterol and less lecithin than those produced by free range chickens. This is because of their limited diet and restricted movements. Make sure that the eggs you eat come only from chickens that can forage freely in the barnyard and that are organically fed. Be aware that some free range chickens are still being fed refined commercial feeds.[7]

Eat foods that are pure and unadulterated. The addition of fertilizers, pesticides, herbicides, additives, artificial

---

[2]Dr. Bernard Jensen, Basic Iridology Seminar, Escondido, CA, 10-28 to 11-01, 1988.
[3]Ibid.
[4]Ibid.
[5]Ibid.
[6]Jensen, *The Chemistry of Man*, p. 276.
[7]Udo Erasmus, *Fats and Oils* (Vancouver, British Columbia: Alive Books, 1986), pp. 227-228.

preservatives, and other human-made chemicals to our food chain has produced several documented examples of harmful side effects. Many people are allergic to these chemical additives without even realizing it.

Consider the type and quality of the foods you are buying. Changing your diet, to become more natural, may mean paying higher prices than you are used to. Still, the value you receive from having a healthier body will be worth it.

35 Practical Ways To Improve Your Health

CHAPTER 26

Rest

Perhaps you know people who are always on the go. From the time they awaken, until the time they go to bed, they are continuously on the run. Maybe you are one of these people.

We find in Genesis 2, verse 1 & 2:

> "Thus the heavens and the earth were finished, and all the host of them. And on the seventh day God ended his work which he had made; and he rested on the seventh day.... And God blessed the seventh day, and sanctified it: because that in it he had rested from all his work which God created and made."

It is not an accident that your Maker set aside one day a week for rest. This was to ensure that you would allow your body enough time to reenergize itself.

Potassium is one of the most difficult minerals for the body to assimilate.[1] It is a necessary nutrient that maintains muscle strength and energy in the body. The best way to increase its assimilation is to do nothing other than rest! The more you can slow down and rest, the more potassium your body can utilize and the healthier you will stay. It's that simple!!

And so it is with all the laws that the God force set in motion for us. When we burn the candle at both ends, we run the risk of burning ourselves up! We wear ourselves out much faster than we should, and this is not what was intended for you and me.

Rest one day a week for your own good! The body needs this time to recharge its energy batteries to allow you to work and play to your maximum for the next six days.

---

[1] Dr. Joseph Manthei, Video Cassette, *Simple Anatomy*, 1985.

35 Practical Ways To Improve Your Health

Now, this does not mean that you work on your lawn and garden, or that you clean your house or run errands. It means to take the day off—period! Use it to spend time with your family or loved ones. Listen to some uplifting music, read a good book, or just relax and contemplate the beauty of the moment. You owe this time to yourself and to others.

CHAPTER 27

Rhythm

You may have the perception that you could make yourself well if only you were eating the right kinds of food. While this would be a sensible approach to improving your health, I believe it is only a part of the story.

Granted, nutrition is an area that is of prime importance, but it is just one of several factors that must be considered. There is more to the making of a healthier body than simply the food we put into it.

For example, let's discuss the role that rhythm plays in your life. We will begin by defining what rhythm is and why it is so important to being healthy.

Rhythm is the daily health routine we follow by performing required body functions throughout certain times of the day. This would include the time we set aside to take a bath or shower, the time we use to shave our legs or face, the time we have our health movements, and the time we take to eat, sleep, work, play, exercise, pray, meditate, etc. It is the daily life pattern we establish for our body.

The more in tune, or the more your body is prepared or expects what will take place during the day, the healthier you will be. For example, people who get sick are usually those who are out of rhythm because their schedule is in chaos, and because they have no order in their life. They eat their evening meals at 9:30 p.m. one night, and 5 p.m. the next. They have breakfast one morning, but not the next.[1]

Rhythm helps to keep the body in harmony. If meals are eaten at a certain time each day, and within a half hour either way, the subconscious body clock can properly

---

[1]Dr. Joseph Manthei, *More Excellent Way Ministries: Home Correspondence Course* (Quarryville, Pennsylvania: by the author, 1978), p. 3.

prepare itself to receive and use these nutrients. This explains why it is not only important to eat the correct foods, but when.[2]

And so it is with every other bodily function. Try to set a routine for all your daily activities and follow it as closely as possible. You'll find you get better results with whatever you are doing.

How did rhythm begin? Look at Genesis, Chapter 1, verses 14-19, the fourth day of creation:

> "And God said, Let there be lights in the firmament of the heaven to divide the day from the night; and let them be for signs, and for seasons, and for days, and years:..... And God made two great lights; the greater light to rule the day, and the lesser light to rule the night: he made the stars also. And God set them in the firmament of the heaven to give light upon the earth, and to rule over the day and over the night, and to divide the light from the darkness: and God saw that it was good."

---

[2]Ibid.

CHAPTER 28

Rice Bran Syrup

Rice bran syrup is composed of concentrated brown rice polishings that are the parts of the whole rice that the miller discards. Rice bran syrup is 17 times stronger than regular rice polishings.[1] It is usually prepared with or without yeast or wheat germ in a malt extract base.

This product is very high in silicon and the B-complex vitamins that are essential nutrients for the nervous system, skin, hair, glands, and nails. It is known that while the rice polishings contain the richest source of silicon,[2] the rice bran syrup, itself, also is the best source of the B-complex vitamins.[3] The polishings provide most, but not all, of the vitamin B-complex. This explains the reason for the syrup's other ingredients, which are used to supply the B-complex vitamins that are missing.

Laboratory experiments, which were conducted to confirm the existence of the B vitamins, involved pigeons that were fed refined white rice. After eating this rice for four days, several pigeons would fall over backward and be dead. Other pigeons, also very near to death, were given the rice polishings and then revived.[4] Some churches today do not allow the throwing of white rice, outside after a wedding, to prevent something similar from happening to any birds or wildlife.

This story illustrates the value in eating only whole foods, and not just portions of it (see Chapter 25). The pigeons needed the silicon and B vitamins that were

---

[1] Bernard Jensen, D.C., Ph.D., *Master Feeding Program* (Escondido, California: by the author, 1988), p. 35.
[2] Dr. Bernard Jensen, Basic Iridology Seminar, Escondido, CA, 10-28 to 11-01, 1988.
[3] Dr. Bernard Jensen, Advanced Iridology Seminar, Escondido, CA, 11-04 to 11-06, 1988.
[4] Bernard Jensen, Ph.D., *The Chemistry of Man* (Escondido, California: by the author, 1983), p. 310.

contained in the outer layers of the rice. The rice bran syrup ensures that you receive the same nutrients.

Caution: This supplement cannot be used by everyone. If you have a tendency toward low blood carbohydrate, do not take it. This is because of the malt extract base.[5]

If you are one of these individuals, do not despair because you can use other foods to receive many of the same benefits. Be sure to eat whole brown rice and wheat germ that can be purchased at most health food or co-op stores. Remember also to drink oat straw tea (see Chapter 15) because it is high in silicon.

Dr. Jensen and Nature's Sunshine Products both carry very fine rice bran syrup products. Dr. Jensen's contains liquid yeast and no wheat germ. Nature's Sunshine product is yeast-free and uses wheat germ instead.

Both syrups have a brown coloring and are semi-sweet tasting. It is recommended to take 1 teaspoonful after every meal. Use the one that fits your diet and health improvement plan the best.

---

[5]Bernard Jensen D.C., *A New Lifestyle for Health & Happiness* (Escondido, California: by the author, 1980), p. 48.

CHAPTER 29

Skin Brushing

The skin is the largest organ of your body. It is unfortunate that it is one that is often overlooked or ignored. Yet a vital and "enlivened" skin is essential to your complete health.[1]

Skin brushing is done to remove the old cells, acids, and mucus that can build up on the surface of the skin. When these are not removed, they interfere with the main function of the skin; that is, to help detoxify the body. This is why I brush my skin every day.

You will need to buy a good vegetable bristle brush at your local health food store or from the recommended vendors shown at the end of this book. Do not purchase or use anything that has a plastic bristle—only natural is acceptable.

Use this before you take your bath or shower. Beginning with your feet and moving up, always brush in a direction toward the center of your body (the colon area). Do not scrub the skin, but move it in a firm and deliberate manner. You want to stimulate it, not scratch or damage it.

After you have finished your legs, start at your hands and move down your arms. Finally, do the neck and chest area, front and back. Do not use the brush on your face. Buy a Loofah brush for that purpose.

---

[1] Dr. Bernard Jensen, Basic Iridology Seminar, Escondido, CA, 10-28 to 11-01, 1988.

35 Practical Ways To Improve Your Health

The brushing action of the skin stimulates the lymphatic system, via the colon, and the surrounding muscles located in the skin to do their job of cleansing toxins from the body. It also will eliminate any dead tissue that is ready to be removed.

The skin is responsible for removing two pounds of toxins from the body a day. Each of the other eliminative organs, such as the colon, lungs and the kidneys, removes the same amount.[2]

In fact, the skin has been called the "third" kidney. Have you ever wondered why on a hot summer day that you need to urinate less than normal although you are drinking more liquids? It is because the skin is helping to remove those toxins, which the kidney would normally handle, by perspiring more.

Look at your skin. Is it vibrant and alive, or does it look pale and sickly? Daily skin brushing can enhance your natural beauty to make sure that it will last as long as you do.

---

[2]Dr. Bernard Jensen, Basic Iridology Seminar, Toronto, Ontario, 06-23 to 06-25, 1989.

CHAPTER 30

Spinal Adjustments

I am a firm believer in chiropractic adjustments. If you have ever had a good chiropractor manipulate your spine when there has been a misalignment, you know what I mean. You definitely feel a lot better.

Keeping the spine in alignment can increase and hold energy in your body. This is very important when you are trying to build optimum health.

There is a belief that a flow of energy moves through your body that is necessary for keeping the organs in your body healthy (see Chapter 32). Dr. Joseph Manthei, a noted chiropractor, explains it this way: "The nervous system associated with the spine controls the muscles.... The vagus nervous system controls the vital organs. Yet there is muscular tissue associated with every vital organ. This is one reason why chiropractors have been successful as they are affecting the muscular tissue associated with the organs and influencing the flow of energy from the brain down through the spinal column and out to the various tissues."[1]

Spinal adjustments are valuable then, because they help keep your back as straight as possible that in turn helps to ensure there are no blockages of this free flow of energy to your muscles and organs.

The chiropractor of today has taken at least six years of highly specialized college training. They must learn more physiology (a branch of biology), neurology (the nervous system), anatomy (the structure of the body), and almost as much chemistry as a medical school graduate. In fact, they must complete more total classroom hours.

---

[1] Dr. Joseph Manthei, *More Excellent Way Ministries: Home Correspondence Course* (Quarryville, Pennsylvania: by the author, 1978), p. 90.

35 Practical Ways To Improve Your Health

Check with your friends to find someone compatible for you. If that doesn't work, as with any professional, use the "yellow pages" of your directory to locate the chiropractor of your choice. There is usually an initial examination, and x-rays could be taken.

CHAPTER 31

Tahini (Sesame Seed Butter)

Sesame is known as the king of the seeds.[1] It is synonymous with strength and though it is one of the smallest seeds we have, it also is one of the most powerful. It has more vitamin E than any other seed and is a rich source of calcium.

In his travels to several foreign countries, Dr. Bernard Jensen determined that the country of Turkey had some of the strongest people in the world. On one occasion, he watched as a 75 year old man carried a piano on his back for nine blocks. He also saw the champion wrestler in Turkey. He too was 75 years old! The sesame seed comprises the base of the halva and tahini foods that are eaten by the Turkish people.[2]

The Turks make a treat from a little sesame seed that is all ground up and dipped in concentrated grape juice; they are then placed on strings to sell or used as candy.[3] It is interesting that grape juice contains the quickest sugar to be absorbed by the body and also is an aid in heart health.

Purchase the raw sesame tahini jar at any health food store. The brand name I use is Westbrae Natural®. Do not buy the toasted sesame seed butter, because heat can alter the nutritional content. It should be raw and organically grown only.

Use at least a tablespoon or more every day. Eat it plain or spread it on bread or crackers for an excellent snack.

---

[1]Dr. Bernard Jensen, 80th Birthday Symposium, San Diego, CA, 08-27 to 09-01, 1988.
[2]Bernard Jensen, D.C., Ph.D., *Master Feeding Program* (Escondido, California: by the author, 1988), p. 32.
[3]Ibid., p. 33.

CHAPTER 32

Thump Your Thymus

The thymus is a small, pinkish-gray, two-lobed endocrine gland located in the center of your upper chest. The full function or purpose of this gland is not completely understood, and information about it is somewhat limited.

Dr. John Diamond has conducted considerable research on the activity and value of the thymus. This chapter is dedicated to the fascinating results of his investigation that he documented in the book *Your Body Doesn't Lie.*

The thymus gland has the important responsibility of keeping our immune system strong. It is the command center for the production and control of lymphocytes or white blood cells. The body uses these cells as a first line of defense against other foreign cells, such as those that are cancerous.

It should be classified as an endocrine gland, similar to the adrenal or pancreas. Here is the reason according to Dr. Diamond: "Lymphocytes, in an immature state, come to the thymus from the bone marrow. Under the influence of thymus hormones, these cells mature, then leave the thymus and settle in the lymph nodes and the spleen, where they give rise to other generations of lymphocytes called T cells (T for thymus-derived). Thymus hormones travel through the bloodstream and continue to exert their influence over the departed T cells. Thus, the thymus can be considered to be a true endocrine gland—that is, an organ that secretes a hormone into the bloodstream to be carried to another part of the body where it will have its effect."[1]

Your current state of health is nothing more than a representation of the amount of usable energy you have

---

[1] Excerpt from *BK: Behavioral Kinesiology*, by John Diamond, M.D., Copyright© 1979 by John Diamond, M.D.

35 Practical Ways To Improve Your Health

available. The thymus is the gland most closely involved with any problems related to this.

You are energy! This is what you consume as you complete your day-to-day activities. It is what you use while you are working, or eating, or sleeping, or thinking, or talking, or whatever. It is a representation of your daily existence on this planet. A higher energy level will help you feel better about yourself. The thymus gland is the key to raising it.

Behavioral kinesiology (BK) is an eclectic approach to treating patients that includes psychosomatic medicine, muscle testing, psychiatry, acupuncture, osteopathy, nutrition and other related sciences. Using BK procedures, it was determined that the thymus played a major role in the amount of energy that can be made available to the body.

The thymus controls what has been denoted as the "Life Energy" center in our bodies. It regulates an internal energy source that is available to everyone, but because of its sensitivity to external pressures, such as stress, needs frequent stimulation.

The way to stimulate it is by thumping your thymus! The thymus is located under the spot where the second rib meets the breastbone (the sternomanubrial joint). This is about four to five inches directly below your Adam's apple (see below).

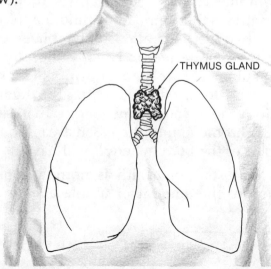

Thump Your Thymus

Make a fist with your hand and then use the flattened portion to thump the thymus area lightly. Rotate your fist (in a *clockwise* direction only), over this area in a circling motion to help stimulate it. This action would be identical, from your viewpoint, to someone standing directly in front of you and moving their fist around you in a similar direction. Continue to do this until you yawn or feel the need to take a deep breath. That's all there is to it!

You now have a simple and easy technique to help raise your body's energy level. You can do this several times a day or whenever you feel your energy level falling.

It is important to mention that additional kinesiology research also is available that claims success in helping to balance the left and right hemispheres of the brain. There are many who believe that the two sides of the brain provide different skill functions. The left is known as the logical, verbal, and rigid side; the right is the artistic, intuitive, and free-flowing side.

The idealized approach to interacting and dealing with life's day-to-day problems would be when both parts of the brain are being used together. This would allow the individual the entire use of their abilities when faced with stressful situations. Unfortunately, BK tests have proven that this is not often the case, since most of us are either left or right brain dominated.

To rectify this, firmly place and hold the tip of your tongue on the roof of your mouth, about 1/4 inch behind your upper front teeth. This action helps to "recenter" or balance your brain activities, which would then assure you of its full use while handling your daily problems.

So, while you are thumping your thymus, remember to hold your tongue in position on your upper mouth. You'll be receiving two benefits simultaneously. I always use this technique during and after my running exercise and feel that it strengthens me. Try it! You will be pleasantly surprised how well it works!

The thymus is very sensitive to stressful conditions. It will weaken when subjected to any of these types of situations. This has a negative effect on the body's ability to fight off diseases and infections.

Thumping your thymus will help ensure that it stays strong so it can regulate the immunological system properly as it was designed for your body. It also will help stabilize and increase your energy level. And what could be better than that?

CHAPTER 33

Unclean Meats

One of the finest authorities on health related issues is the Bible. It's true. The Creator left nothing to chance. He mandated His laws on cleanliness, through the myriad of chapters of the Old and New Testaments, to be sure that we would not do harm to ourselves through a careless diet.

You can read about several of these laws, as discussed in Leviticus, Chapter 11, which relate to unclean red meats, fish, or fowl. Verses 1 through 11 are presented below:

"And the Lord spake unto Moses and to Aaron, saying unto them, speak unto the children of Israel, saying, These are the beasts which ye shall eat among all the beasts that are on the earth. Whatsoever parteth the hoof, and is clovenfooted, and cheweth the cud, among the beasts, that shall ye eat. Nevertheless these shall ye not eat of them that chew the cud, or of them that divide the hoof: as the camel, because he cheweth the cud, but divideth not the hoof; he is unclean to you.... And the swine [hog -Ed.], though he divide the hoof, and be clovenfooted, yet he cheweth not the cud; he is unclean to you. Of their flesh shall ye not eat,....

"These shall ye eat of all that are in the waters: whatsoever hath fins and scales in the waters, in the seas, and in the rivers, them shall ye eat. And all that have not fins and scales in the seas, and in the rivers, of all that move in the waters, and of any living thing which is in the waters, they shall be an abomination unto you:...; ye shall not eat of their flesh,...."

Deuteronomy, Chapter 14, also addresses this subject.

35 Practical Ways To Improve Your Health

It is clear what our Maker had in mind when these laws were given. Only certain types of meat would be compatible with the human body. That would include beef, lamb, deer, buffalo, elk, chicken, turkey, etc., and only fish with fins or scales such as salmon and herring. Consequently, this would rule out meats such as pork, goose, duck, tuna, catfish, shrimp, lobsters, clams, oysters, etc., that are not compatible.

Unclean meats release their energy too quickly during the digestion process, and the body cannot use it properly. These meats age the body prematurely.[1] You would do well to leave them alone.

If you eat the clean meats, it is a good idea to soak them in cold salt water for about 12 hours, then rinse and replace in clean water for another 24. This preparation draws the blood from the meat and enhances the quality of it. This is called "koshering" within the Jewish religion. Try this! You'll taste the difference!

You can make your own decision about what foods are acceptable to eat, but I believe that the laws that the God force set in motion during the Old Testament are as valid today as they were then. When we break these laws, we reduce our chances of ever reaching our best health potential.

---

[1] Carey A. Reams with Cliff Dudley, *Choose Life or Death* (Harrison, Arkansas: New Leaf Press, Inc., 1978), p. 59.

CHAPTER 34

Vitamin "E" & Lecithin

The human brain is the most important organ in the body. It is responsible for the proper functioning of every other organ. It needs four times as much oxygen as the other areas of the body.[1] When the brain dies, the body dies.

The brain and the extremities (hands and feet) are those parts of the body that are the farthest from the heart, and accordingly, most difficult to nourish. Because of this, it makes it hard for nutrients to reach these vital portions.

The heart has the very unenviable job of pumping blood and oxygen, against gravity, to the brain area that is directly above it. Therefore, it is beneficial for your health to help or increase this flow of oxygen to the brain.

Vitamin E and lecithin (see Chapter 25) can do that. Vitamin E brings four times as much oxygen to the head.[2] It does this by thinning the blood, which in turn allows it to hold more oxygen.[3] The thinner the blood, the easier it is for the heart to pump it. Is it any wonder then that vitamin E is known as the "heart" vitamin?

Lecithin dissolves cholesterol. This action helps ensure that the circulatory system is kept clean and open, while it provides a more consistent flow of blood and nutrients throughout the body, and places less strain on the heart muscle.

Almost everyone over the age of 45 should be taking lecithin and vitamin E.[4] They are very helpful for those people with heart conditions.

---

[1] Dr. Bernard Jensen, 80th Birthday Symposium, 08-27 to 09-01, 1988.
[2] Ibid.
[3] Dr. Joseph Manthei, *More Excellent Way Ministries: Home Correspondence Course* (Quarryville, Pennsylvania: by the author, 1978), p. 78.
[4] Dr. Bernard Jensen, Basic Iridology Seminar, Toronto, Ontario, 06-23 to 06-25, 1989.

In addition, lecithin also is a fat that is needed by the brain and nerves,[5] and certain types are a good source of the essential fatty acids (see Chapters 4, 14, & 25).[6] Vitamin E also has been used effectively for varicose vein problems.[7]

Check with your doctor first, but it should be safe to take between 400 and 800 International Units (I.U.) of vitamin E a day. Be sure to purchase only the natural kind. The label will say "contains natural d-Alpha Tocopherol...." This is the one you should use. If it shows an "l," such as "dl-Alpha Tocopheryl Acetate," or says "d-Alpha Tocopheryl Acetate," it means it is of a synthetic kind. Pass it by.

NatureMost® Laboratories Inc. (see the Recommended Vendor List) produces an excellent vitamin E capsule that is available in 400 I.U. strength. It also contains lecithin.

Much of the lecithin on the market today is manufactured from soybean oil because it contains both the omega 3 and omega 6 essential fatty acids, unlike many other seeds containing only the omega 6, and it is inexpensive to produce. You can buy it at most nutrition stores. I use capsules from Nature's Sunshine Products. Again, discuss this with your doctor before you start using it.

Caution!! If you have or even suspect a heart condition, you must be very careful when using lecithin! Because of its affinity for cholesterol there is always the chance that a piece could break free and clog a major artery. Use it only under the direct consultation of your physician!

It is possible that the addition of a lipase fat digestive aid (see Chapter 11), for use with the lecithin, would then be necessary. For all others, take as directed on the bottle.

---

[5]Dr. Bernard Jensen, Basic Iridology Seminar, Escondido, CA, 10-28 to 11-01, 1988.
[6]Udo Erasmus, *Fats and Oils* (Vancouver, British Columbia: Alive Books, 1986), pp. 55-56.
[7]Dr. Bernard Jensen, Basic Iridology Seminar, Toronto, Ontario, 06-23 to 06-25, 1989.

CHAPTER 35

Wheat & Milk Allergies

Many of us are allergic to different foods without even realizing it. There is a belief that for most every food that exists, someone is allergic to it.[1]

A common source of allergies, for children or adults, is wheat and milk products. So common, in fact, that many doctors will test these two foods first when checking for allergies because they are so prevalent.

One type of allergic reaction to cow's milk will produce a profuse diarrhea. It is the protein in the milk that causes this allergy. Many babies become allergic to milk because their digestive systems are not designed to handle this type of food.

There is an excellent substitute that can be used instead: raw goat's milk (see Chapter 24). There will be very few children who are allergic to goat's milk, as it is the most closely related milk, chemically speaking, to a nursing mother's. It has little mucus and is very low in fat.

Adults can use it also as it is very nutritious. It is a favorite of Dr. Bernard Jensen for his patients because he says it is a food that feeds the whole body. Almost everyone would benefit from using it.

Wheat allergies might appear as sinus, bronchial, or asthma conditions. Wheat can cause other problems also because of its high gluten content (it doesn't matter if it is the whole or refined version). Gluten is the "glue" or sticky substance that holds the bread together when you are preparing it.

---

[1] Carey A. Reams with Cliff Dudley, *Choose Life or Death* (Harrison, Arkansas: New Leaf Press, Inc., 1978), p. 119.

Gluten breaks down the minute villi in the small intestine where the absorption from digesting food takes place. Without these important villi, the body is unable to extract the nutrition that it must have. There is even a name for this condition; it is known as celiac disease.

Millet is a good substitute for wheat because it contains no gluten. Yale University conducted a study on dogs that addressed the differences associated with diets that were high in either wheat or millet. One control group ate nothing but wheat products, the other millet.

The former group was lethargic, with a very low energy level, and they had become fat. The dogs in the millet test group were frisky, energetic and lean.[2]

Millet is a rich food source of vitamin B-17. This also is called amygdalin, or perhaps you know it better by its other name: laetrile.

Some of the world's finest Olympic running and skiing champions are from the Scandinavian countries. Dr. Jensen believes it is because of another low gluten food that is so prevalent in their diet: rye. This has prompted him to make these statements: "Rye builds muscle. Wheat builds fat."[3]

Present-day wheat is a hybrid grain; rye is an original. One has been crossbred by humankind, its composition significantly changed to increase the gluten content, while the other has remained much closer to its native state as originally found and harvested on this planet. Is it possible a Source higher than ourselves knew which foods were better for us than we did, or is that just a coincidence?

There are two other good substitutions you can use for the wheat as well.[4] They are yellow cornmeal, one of the richest magnesium sources available (see related Chapter 10), and whole brown rice (see related Chapter 28). Both have little or no gluten. These two grains, including the

---

[2]Bernard Jensen, D.C., Ph. D., *Master Feeding Program* (Escondido, California: by the author, 1988), p. 29.
[3]Ibid.
[4]Ibid.

Wheat & Milk Allergies

millet and rye, also are high in calcium.

There are several ways to prepare these grains, which should be bought organically grown whenever possible. Here is just one method.

For the whole grain millet, brown rice, and rye:

Use 2 1/2 parts water to 1 part grain (this proportion can vary depending on your preference for thickness).

For the ground yellow cornmeal:

Use 3 to 4 parts water to 1 part grain (this proportion can vary depending on your preference for thickness).

Bring the water to a boil in a stainless steel pan which has a lid.

Add the grain, turn the heat to low, stirring occasionally, and cook for around 45 minutes (15 to 20 minutes for the yellow cornmeal).

Raw honey can be used to sweeten the cereal.

35 Practical Ways To Improve Your Health

Dr. Jensen is deeply interested in improving the health of this country. He's concerned about a study that claimed that up to 62% of the average American diet consisted of the following food groups (see chart below):[5]

Wheat or Gluten Products	29%
Milk Products	25%
Sugar	06 - 08%

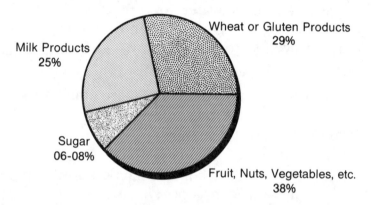

That leaves only 38% of the diet available for other nutrition sources. How close do these figures match your diet?

You are an end result of the foods that you are choosing to eat or drink. While it would be very difficult to eliminate all wheat and milk products completely, at least consider reducing the amount because of the allergies or problems they can cause. This will leave room in your diet for other foods, such as the raw goat's milk or millet, which could be the key to improving your health.

---

[5] Ibid., p. 25.

Happy and Healthy, Naturally...

I believe the best way to improve your health is by following a lifestyle that cares for the whole body instead of just individual organs. Many nutritional or holistic practices described in this book will do just that. They all work together to ensure that we stay happy and healthy, naturally...

Here is a listing of the body systems and nutritive areas that are supported by my program, followed by their corresponding chapter(s):

Brain:	Vitamin E & Lecithin; Raw, Whole, & Pure (Egg Yolk); Exercise; Bee Pollen (Rutin); Niacin Flush; Rest; Raw Goat's Milk
Thymus:	Thump Your Thymus; Herbal Teas (Oatstraw, Horsetail)
Thyroid:	Iodine; Herbal Teas (Oatstraw, Horsetail)
Heart:	Vitamin E & Lecithin; Herbal Teas (Hawthorn Berry); Exercise; Rest; Potato Peeling Broth
Liver:	Herbal Teas (Dandelion); Distilled Water
Gall Bladder:	Herbal Teas (Dandelion)
Pancreas:	Chlorophyll
Spleen:	Herbal Teas (Pau D'Arco); Raw Goat's Milk
Stomach:	Raw Goat's Milk; Aloe Vera; Alfalfa Tablets; Cayenne Pepper

35 Practical Ways To Improve Your Health

Colon:	Cleanse Your Colon; Herbal Teas (Flaxseed); Flaxseed; Aloe Vera; Alfalfa Tablets; Rainbow-Colored Salads; Potato Peeling Broth; Rhythm; Exercise; Liquid Minerals
Small Intestine:	Herbal Teas (Flaxseed); Aloe Vera
Kidneys:	Herbal Teas (Horsetail, Cornsilk, Uva Ursi); Distilled Water; Potato Peeling Broth
Bladder:	Herbal Teas (Horsetail, Cornsilk, Uva Ursi); Distilled Water
Lungs:	All Spices & Herbs (ASH); Liquid Minerals; Exercise
Bones:	Herbal Teas (Comfrey); Min-Col; Wheat & Milk Allergies (Rye, Millet, Yellow Cornmeal, Whole Brown Rice); Raw Goat's Milk; Sesame Seed Butter
Skin:	Herbal Teas (Oatstraw, Horsetail); Skin Brushing; Bee Pollen; Rice Bran Syrup; Flaxseed
Teeth, Nails:	Herbal Teas (Oatstraw, Horsetail); Min-Col; Rice Bran Syrup; Alfalfa Tablets
Hair:	Herbal Teas (Oatstraw, Horsetail); Rice Bran Syrup; Flaxseed
Glands:	Herbal Teas (Oatstraw, Horsetail); Bee Pollen; Rice Bran Syrup; Sesame Seed Butter; Flaxseed; Iodine
Joints:	Raw Goat's Milk; Exercise
Immune System:	Herbal Teas (Pau D'Arco); Thump Your Thymus; Raw Goat's Milk; Rest
Nervous System:	Spinal Adjustments; Herbal Teas (Oatstraw, Horsetail, Peppermint); Rice Bran Syrup; Raw, Whole, & Pure (Egg Yolk); Rest; Flaxseed; Raw Goat's Milk

Skeletal System:	Sesame Seed Butter; Raw Goat's Milk; Spinal Adjustments; Min-Col; Herbal Teas (Comfrey); Wheat & Milk Allergies (Rye, Millet, Yellow Corn Meal, Whole Brown Rice); Exercise
Respiratory System:	Exercise; Liquid Minerals; All Spices & Herbs (ASH)
Lymphatic System:	Raw Goat's Milk; Distilled Water; Skin Brushing; Exercise
Circulation System:	Niacin Flush; Herbal Teas (Hawthorn Berry); Vitamin E & Lecithin; Chlorophyll; Exercise; Cayenne Pepper; Distilled Water; Alfalfa Tablets; Rainbow-Colored Salads (Red & Green Vegetables); Potato Peeling Broth
Digestive System:	Digestive Aids; Liquid Minerals; Rhythm; Bee Pollen; Raw, Whole, & Pure; Distilled Water; Herbal Teas (Peppermint, Alfalfa); Rainbow-Colored Salads; Aloe Vera; Raw Goat's Milk; Cayenne Pepper
Elimination System:	Cleanse Your Colon; Flaxseed; Alfalfa Tablets; Rhythm; Skin Brushing; Distilled Water; Herbal Teas (Alfalfa, Flaxseed, Dandelion, Horsetail, Uva Ursi, Cornsilk); Aloe Vera; Wheat & Milk Allergies (Yellow Corn Meal); Rainbow-Colored Salads; Potato Peeling Broth; Raw, Whole, & Pure; Exercise; Liquid Minerals
Reproductive System:	Herbal Teas (Red Raspberry - Women)
Muscular System:	Exercise; Potato Peeling Broth; Wheat & Milk Allergies (Rye); Spinal Adjustments; Raw Goat's Milk

35 Practical Ways To Improve Your Health

Glandular System:	Iodine; Herbal Teas (Oatstraw, Horsetail); Sesame Seed Butter; Bee Pollen; Rice Bran Syrup; Unclean Meats (Premature Aging)
Spiritual:	Belief in Someone Higher Than You; Change Your Attitude; Learn To Love
Emotional:	Learn To Love; Rest
Energy:	Bee Pollen; Cayenne Pepper; Thump Your Thymus; Exercise; Rest; Spinal Adjustments; Distilled Water; Sesame Seed Butter; Liquid Minerals
General Body Builder:	Chlorophyll; Liquid Minerals; Raw Goat's Milk; Raw, Whole, & Pure (Egg Yolk); Rainbow-Colored Salads; Bee Pollen; Min-Col; Blackstrap Molasses; Alfalfa Tablets; Exercise; All Spices & Herbs (ASH); Cleanse Your Colon
Vitamin A:	Rainbow-Colored Salads (Orange & Yellow Vegetables); Bee Pollen
Vitamin B-Complex:	Rice Bran Syrup; Wheat & Milk Allergies (Rye, Millet, Yellow Cornmeal, Whole Brown Rice); Bee Pollen
Vitamin C:	Onion Soup; Bee Pollen
Vitamin D:	Alfalfa Tablets; Bee Pollen
Vitamin E:	Vitamin E & Lecithin (Supplement); Sesame Seed Butter; Bee Pollen
Vitamin F: (Essential Fatty Acids)	Flaxseed; Bee Pollen; Raw, Whole, & Pure (Egg Yolk); Sesame Seed Butter; Vitamin E & Lecithin
Vitamin K:	Chlorophyll; Alfalfa Tablets
Vitamin P:	Bee Pollen (Rutin)
Vitamin U:	Alfalfa Tablets

Essential Amino Acids:	Alfalfa Tablets; Flaxseed; Bee Pollen; Raw, Whole, & Pure (Egg Yolk)
Lecithin:	Aloe Vera; Bee Pollen; Vitamin E & Lecithin; Raw, Whole, & Pure (Egg Yolk)
Calcium:	Wheat & Milk Allergies (Rye, Millet, Yellow Cornmeal, Whole Brown Rice); Raw Goat's Milk; Rainbow-Colored Salads; Herbal Teas (Comfrey); Min-Col; Sesame Seed Butter
Potassium:	Potato Peeling Broth; Blackstrap Molasses; Rest; Alfalfa Tablets; Aloe Vera; Raw Goat's Milk
Silicon:	Herbal Teas (Oatstraw, Horsetail); Flaxseed; Alfalfa Tablets; Rice Bran Syrup
Sodium:	Raw Goat's Milk; Liquid Minerals; Alfalfa Tablets; Aloe Vera
Iodine:	Iodine (Kelp, Dulse); Liquid Minerals
Iron:	Blackstrap Molasses; Chlorophyll (Black Cherry Juice)
Phosphorus:	Raw, Whole, & Pure (Egg Yolk); Raw Goat's Milk
Magnesium:	Alfalfa Tablets; Wheat & Milk Allergies (Yellow Corn Meal); Liquid Minerals; Aloe Vera
Manganese:	Iodine (Dulse); Rainbow-Colored Salads (Vegetables with Seeds)
Fluorine:	Raw Goat's Milk; Min-Col
Trace Minerals:	Alfalfa Tablets; Liquid Minerals; Blackstrap Molasses; Bee Pollen

Epilogue: The Healing Crisis

Many of us are interested in becoming more healthy. I have included the previous chapters to help you do that. Yet, it was not my intention for you to think that this process would be easy. I did try, however, to include information that would make the change easier, and there is a difference.

If you are patient and diligent about following the ideas mentioned in this book, you should notice an improvement in your health. As this occurs, your body is going to start changing for the better. You may even go through what is called a "healing crisis."

The person who first indentified the healing crisis was a homeopathic doctor by the name of Hering.[1] Hering's *Law of Cure*, which it became known as, was used by him to explain the health changes that his patients experienced.

It consisted of the following three parts:

> "All cure starts from within out and from the head down and in reverse order as the symptoms have appeared."[2]

Thus, you renew yourself, first, from the inside out, starting with the head area and moving downward, and then you will reexperience any previous changes in the level of your health.

This means that the fever you once had as a child, which was suppressed, may reappear. Other significant physical or emotional changes in your health, that have occurred to you in the past, also could surface.

---

[1] Bernard Jensen, D.C., *Doctor-Patient Handbook* (Escondido, California: Bernard Jensen Enterprises, 1976), p. III.
[2] Ibid., p. 54.

It will happen when the body has rebuilt itself to the point where it can now push out the old, toxic cells and replace them with new, healthier ones. It is actually a cleansing process that is taking place in the body. I want to assure you that this is not happening because of something you have done wrong. It is the real reward for all your hard work!

The healing crisis will last anywhere from about three days to two weeks. Make yourself as comfortable as possible during this process, and remember that it too, will pass. Most people will comment about how good they are feeling before the beginning of a healing crisis. It will be helpful to take the potato peeling broth (see Chapter 22) during this period.

The healing crisis is more thoroughly documented in Dr. Jensen's excellent book *Doctor-Patient Handbook*. Do yourself a favor and purchase a copy.

Recommended Vendor List

Bernard Jensen International
24360 Old Wagon Rd.
Escondido, California 92027
(619) 749-2727

Product	Size	Price* (subject to change)
Alfalfa Tablets	500	$ 4.05
	1000	7.43
Chlorophyll	pint	6.95
Colon Cleansing Program	—	60.00 (approx.)
Liquid Dulse (Iodine)	1 oz.	1.75
	4 oz.	5.95
Rice Bran Syrup	pint	7.90
Skin Brush	—	3.75
Whex®	12 oz.	16.00

C C Pollen Company
3627 E. Indian School Road
Suite 209
Phoenix, Arizona 85018-5126
1-800-875-0096 (Toll Free)

Product	Size	Price* (subject to change)
High Desert® Honeybee	1 lb.	$ 15.00
PollenS™ (granules)	5 lb.	70.00
The President's Lunch™ Bar	1.3 oz.	.90

*Effective date 3-1-92.

Cornucopia Specialty Shoppe
Dr. Joseph Manthei
853 Scotland Road
Quarryville, Pennsylvania 17566
(717) 284-3181

Product	Size	Price*
		(subject to change)
All Spices & Herbs (ASH)	1.1 oz. (shaker)	$ 6.00
	1/2 lb. bulk	17.00
	1 lb. bulk	30.00
Min-Col (capsules)	250	18.50
Help From the Sanctuary (food preparation manual)		15.95
More Excellent Way Ministries: Home Correspondence Course		Send for information

Enzymes International, Inc.
P.O. Box 157
Manitowish Waters, Wisconsin 54545
(715) 543-8401

Product	Size	Price*
		(subject to change)
Digestive Aids		
Food Enzymes (capsules)	200	$ 17.00
Hydrochloric Acid (HCl)		
(capsules)	200	15.50
Papaya - Green		
(tablets)	180	19.00
(powder)	8 oz.	32.00
Liquid Coenzyme Minerals	quart	11.50
	gallon	34.50

*Effective date 3-1-92.

Recommended Vendor List

Happy and Healthy, Naturally...
Reid Lassonde
8124 33rd Place North
Crystal, Minnesota 55427
(612) 544-5471

Product	Size	Price*
		(subject to change)
Stainless Steel Water Distillers Pure Water, Inc. - Midi Still D™		$499.00†

†Bottled distilled water costs between $.39 & $1.00. You can distill yours for about $.25/gallon.

Marine Minerals
1990 West 3300 South
Ogden, Utah 84401
1-800-444-8077 (Toll Free)

Product	Size	Price*
		(subject to change)
Liquid Trace Minerals	8 oz.	$ 14.55

Natural Ovens of Manitowoc, Wisconsin
Manitowoc, Wisconsin 54221-2137
1-800-558-3535 (Toll Free)

Product

Flaxseed Breads and Energy Drinks

*Effective date 3-1-92.

NatureMost® Laboratories Inc.
P. O. Box 721
Middletown, Connecticut 06457
(203) 346-8991

Product	Size	Price*
		(subject to change)
Niacin (100 mg. tablets)	250	$ 5.20
Vitamin E (with Lecithin)	100 (400 I.U.)	11.00

Nature's Sunshine Products
P. O. Box 1000
Spanish Fork, Utah 84660
1-800-453-1422 (Toll Free)

Product	Size	Price*
		(subject to change)
Alfalfa (capsules)	100	$ 7.50
	270	20.20
Aloe Vera Juice	quart	13.95
	gallon	44.45
Cayenne Pepper (capsules)	100	7.40
	270	19.95
Chlorophyll	pint	9.45
	quart	17.85
Digestive Aids		
Food Enzymes (tablets) (HCl & Pepsin incl.)	200	25.60
PDA Combination (tablets) (Hydrochloric Acid (HCl) & Pepsin, no Food Enzymes)	200	12.80
Papaya (tablets)	70	7.30
Lecithin (capsules)	270	16.75
Rice Bran Syrup (no yeast)	pint	14.70
Ten Day Colon Cleansing Program		25.70

*Effective date 3-1-92.

Bibliography

Armstrong, Herbert W. *Did God Create a Devil?* Pasadena, California: Worldwide Church of God, 1978.

Armstrong, Herbert W. *Mystery of the Ages.* Pasadena, California: Worldwide Church of God, 1985.

Banik, Dr., Allen E. *The Choice Is Clear.* Kansas City, Missouri: Acres U.S.A., 1975.

Brown, Royden. *How to Live the Millennium: The Bee Pollen Bible.* Phoenix, Arizona: Plains Corporation, 1989.

Diamond, M.D., John. *BK: Behavioral Kinesiology.* New York: Harper & Row, 1979.

Dougherty, Esther. *You Have a Right to Know.* rev. ed. Lincoln, Nebraska: Kane Associates, 1980.

Erasmus, Udo. *Fats and Oils.* Vancouver, British Columbia: Alive Books, 1986.

Gentet, Robert E. *Dinosaurs Before Adam?* Pasadena, California: Ambassador College, 1972.

Gray, Robert. *The Colon Health Handbook.* 6th ed. Oakland, California: Rockridge Publishing Company, 1982.

Holy Bible: King James Version. Cleveland, Ohio: The World Publishing Company.

Howard, Dr., A. B. *Herbal Extracts.* Berkley, Michigan: The Blue Goose Press, 1983.

Is Honeybee Pollen the World's Only Perfect Food? Phoenix, Arizona: C C Pollen Company, 1984.

Jarvis, M.D., D.C. *Folk Medicine.* New York: Fawcett Crest Books, 1958.

Jensen, Ph.D., Bernard. *The Chemistry of Man.* Escondido, California: by the author, 1983.

Jensen, Dr., Bernard. *Creating a Magic Kitchen.* Escondido, California: Bernard Jensen Enterprises, 1973.

Jensen, D.C., Bernard. *Doctor-Patient Handbook.* Escondido, California: Bernard Jensen Enterprises, 1976.

Jensen, D.C., Ph.D., Bernard. *Master Feeding Program.* Escondido, California: by the author, 1988.

Jensen, Bernard. *Nature Has a Remedy.* Escondido, California: by the author, 1978.

Jensen, D.C., Bernard. *A New Lifestyle for Health & Happiness.* Escondido, California: by the author, 1980.

Jensen, D.C., Bernard. *Tissue Cleansing Through Bowel Management.* Escondido, California: by the author, 1980.

Manthei, D.C., Joseph C. *Health Through Diet.* Quarryville, Pennsylvania: More Excellent Way Ministries, 1983.

Manthei, Dr., Joseph. *More Excellent Way Ministries: Diet Booklet.* Quarryville, Pennsylvania: by the author, 1978.

Manthei, Dr., Joseph. *More Excellent Way Ministries: Home Correspondence Course.* Quarryville, Pennsylvania: by the author, 1978.

Manthei, Pamela S. *Help From the Sanctuary.* USA: by the author, 1985.

Muehling, Eldon C. *Water for the Eighties: A Cause for Concern.* Lincoln, Nebraska: Kane Associates, 1979.

Reams, Carey A. with Cliff Dudley. *Choose Life or Death.* Harrison, Arkansas: New Leaf Press, Inc., 1978.

Royal, Penny C. *Herbally Yours.* 3rd ed. Provo, Utah: Sound Nutrition, 1982.

Stitt, M.S., Paul. *The Power of Flax* (pamphlet).

A Systems Guide to Natural Health. Spanish Fork, Utah: Nature's Sunshine Products, Inc., 1988.

Tenney, Louise. *Today's Herbal Health.* 2nd ed. Provo, Utah: Woodland Books, 1983.

Walker, D.Sc., Ph.D., Norman W. *Colon Health: The Key to a Vibrant Life.* Prescott, Arizona: Norwalk Press, 1979.

Index

A
Aaron, 109
Acerola cherries, 79
Acidophilus, 43
Acids, 45, 50, 81, 99
Adam & Eve, 72
Adam's apple, 106
Adrenals, 105
Aging, 22, 110
Alfalfa, 15-16, 36, 41, 59
   digestive enzymes, 15
   essential amino acids, 15
   "father of all foods," 15
Alfalfa tablets, 15-16, 41
Alfalfa tea, 59
All Spices & Herbs (ASH), 17-18, 80
Allantoin, 20
   aloe vera, 20
   comfrey, 20, 58
Allergies, 17, 23, 41, 43, 85-87, 91, 113-116
   bee pollen, 23
   chemicals, 91
   milk, 85-87, 113
   wheat, 113
Aloe vera, 19-20
   gel, 19-20
   "healing" plant, 19
   juice, 19-20
Aluminum, 15
Amino acids, 22, 46, 49
Amygdalin, 114
Amylase, 45
Anal sphincter muscle, 39, 42
Anatomy, 101

Anemia, 35
Angels, 72-73
Antigens, 48
Antiseptic, 22
Anus, 39
Appendix, 39
   lubricates ileo-cecal valve, 39
   "oil can," 39
Arginine, 46
Arms, 99
Armstrong, Herbert W., 73
Artery, 112
Arthritis, 81
Ascending colon, 39
Asthma, 113
Atomic weight, 67
Attitude, 25, 31-33

B
Bacteria, 22, 43, 47, 50, 88
Bananas, 42
Banik, Dr. Allen E., 49
Barley, 80
Basil, 79
Beans, 42, 83
Beaumont, Dr. William, 29
Bee pollen, 21-23
   essential amino acids, 22
   essential fatty acids, 22
   feeds the whole body, 22
   nature's perfect food, 22
Beef, 110
Beets, 83
Behavioral kinesiology, 106-107
Belief systems, 25, 32
Bentonite, 43
Bib lettuce, 83

35 Practical Ways To Improve Your Health

Bible, 72, 109
Birds, 97
Black cherry juice, 35
Black tea, 59
Blackstrap molasses, 18, 27-28, 80, 86-87
Bladder, 59
Bleeding, 29
Blood, 35, 41, 48, 51-52, 68, 77, 110-111
Blood builder, 35, 83
   red & green vegetables, 83
   tonic, 36
Blood capillaries, 22, 77
Blood clotting, 15, 16
Blood plasma, 68
Blood platelets, 55
Blood pressure, 29
Blood purifier, 59
Blood vessels, 77
Bloodstream, 105
Body heat, 61
Bone marrow, 105
Bone meal, 71, 73-74
Bones, 58, 71-72, 74, 85, 87
Bottled water, 48
Bowel, 16, 37, 39, 41-43, 53, 75
   gas, 42-43
Bowel movement, 40-41
Brain, 51, 77, 87, 101, 107, 111-112
Bread, 42, 54, 103, 113
   gluten, 113-114, 116
Breastbone, 106
Broccoli, 83
Bronchial condition, 113
Broth, 81-82
Broth powder, 79-80
Brown rice, 89, 114-115
Brown rice polishings, 97
Brown, Royden, 21
Buffalo, 110
Bulk, 16, 41, 54

Burns, 19

C

C C Pollen Company, 22
Cabbage, 83
Calcium, 15, 20, 22, 30, 42, 53, 58, 61, 71, 85-87, 103, 115
Camel, 109
Cancer, 64, 105
Capillaries, 22, 77
Capsicum, 29-30
Carbohydrates, 45
Carbon, 67
Carbonated beverages, 20
Carrots, 61, 81, 83
Cartilage, 46
Cascara Sagrada, 42
Casseroles, 18, 30
Catfish, 110
Cauliflower, 27, 83
Cayenne pepper, 29-30
Cecum, 37, 39
Celery, 81, 83
Celiac disease, 114
Cells, 20, 49, 59, 69, 99, 105, 124
Cellular level, 67
Cellulase, 45
Cereal, 54
Change your attitude, 31-33, 44
Chard, 83
Cheese, 87
Chelate, 68
Chelated minerals, 67-68
Chemicals, 47, 74, 91
Chemistry, 71, 80, 101
Chest, 21, 99, 105
Chicken, 90, 110
Chiropractor, 101-102
Chlorine, 15
Chlorophyll, 15, 35-36, 84
Chocolate, 59
Cholesterol, 90, 111-112

Index

Circulation, 29, 77
Circulatory system, 35, 58, 111
Clams, 110
Clean meats, 110
    beef, 110
    buffalo, 110
    chicken, 110
    deer, 110
    elk, 110
    herring, 110
    lamb, 110
    salmon, 110
    turkey, 110
Cold-pressed oils, 55
Colds, 79
Coliform bacteria, 43
Collagen, 79
Colloid, 68
Colloidal minerals, 68, 71, 74-75
Colon, 16, 20, 21, 37-44, 54, 99-100
    anal sphincter muscle, 39, 42
    anus, 39
    appendix, 39
    ascending, 39
    bulk (fiber), 16, 41, 54
    cecum, 37, 39
    descending, 39
    hepatic flexure, 39
    ileo-cecal valve, 37, 39
    lubrication, 41-42, 54
    peristalsis action, 42
    rectum, 39
    sigmoid, 39
    sigmoid flexure, 39
    splenic flexure, 39
    transverse, 39
Colon cleansing program, 43-44
Color, 19, 35, 42, 46, 83-84
Comfrey tea, 20, 58
Condiments, 17, 27, 30, 61
Constipation, 40, 42-43, 53-54
Contaminant, 47-48

Cooked foods, 89
    how to prepare, 89
Corinthians, 72
Cornsilk tea, 59
Cottage cheese, 87
Cow, 73, 85
Cow bones, 73
Cow's milk, 85
Crackers, 103
Cranberry juice, 50
Cream, 43
Creator, 25, 31, 37, 109
Cucumbers, 83
Cuts, 19

D

Dandelion tea, 59
David, 26
Deer, 35, 110
Deodorizer, 35
Descending colon, 39
Deuteronomy, 88, 109
Diamond, Dr. John, 105
Diarrhea, 40, 42-43, 53, 68, 113
Digestion, 16, 20, 37, 46, 68, 84, 110, 114
Digestion system, 29, 42, 45, 58-59, 89, 113
Digestive aids, 45-46, 112
    food enzymes, 45-46
    hydrochloric acid (HCl), 45-46
    papaya, 46
Digestive enzymes, 15, 46
Digestive juices, 46
DHA, 54
Dinosaurs, 71-74
Disease, 108
Distillation, 47-48
Distilled water, 20, 36, 47-50, 53, 57, 69, 79, 82
    "catalyst" for new cells, 49
    doesn't "leach out" minerals, 49

drinking guidelines, 49
nature's hydrological cycle, 48
pure, 49-50
Diuretic, 59
Diverticula, 16, 40-41
Diverticulitis, 40-41
Diverticulosis, 40
Diverticulum, 40
DNA, 46
Dogs, 114
Dougherty, Esther, 48
Duck, 110
Dulse, 62

E
Ears, 79
Eggplant, 80
Eggs, 18, 90
  how to prepare, 90
Egg yolk, 90
  essential amino acids, 90
  essential fatty acids, 90
  feeds the whole body, 90
Eisenhower's doctor, Dwight, 51
Electrical energy, 69
Electrolytes, 69
Electron, 67
Elimination system, 16, 20, 39, 42-43, 49, 53-54, 59, 100
Elk, 110
Emotional, 31, 64-65, 123
Endocrine gland, 105
Energy, 22, 25, 29, 31, 35, 49, 52, 61, 63-64, 67, 93, 101, 105-108, 110, 114
Enzymes, 45-46
Enzymes International, Inc., 46, 68-69
EPA, 54
Erasmus, Udo, 15-16, 55, 90, 112
Eskimo, 54-55
Essential amino acids, 15, 22, 55, 90
  isoleucine, 15

leucine, 15
lysine, 15-16
methionine, 15
phenylalanine, 15
threonine, 15
tryptophan, 15-16
valine, 15
Essential fatty acids, 22, 53-55, 90, 112
  linoleic acid, 54
    omega 6, 42, 54, 112
  linolenic acid, 54
    omega 3, 42, 54, 112
Exercise, 41, 46, 51-52, 107
  walking, 51-52
Extremities, 77, 111

F
Face, 99
Fat, 45-46, 55, 112-114
Fat globule, 87
Fatigue, 61
Fear, 35
  acid, 35
Fecal matter, 40-41, 43
Fecal pockets, 16
Feet, 74, 99, 111
Female organs, 59
Fever, 81, 123
Fiber, 16, 41, 43, 45
Fish, 54, 109-110
Fist, 107
Flaxseed, 42, 53-55
  essential amino acids, 55
  essential fatty acids, 53-55
Flaxseed tea, 42, 53, 57-58
  how to prepare, 53
Fluorine, 71, 87
Fluoride, 15
Food digestive enzymes, 22, 45-46, 68, 89
  amylase, 45

Index

cellulase, 45
lipase, 45, 112
protease, 45
Foot, 52
Fowl, 109
Fruits, 41, 49, 79, 116

G
Gall bladder, 59
Garlic, 17
Gas, 42, 46, 84
Gastrointestinal tract, 53
Gelatin, 41
Genesis, 72-73, 75, 93, 96
Gentet, Robert E., 72
Germicidal fluid, 39
Glands, 22, 53, 58, 97, 105-106
Gluten, 113-114, 116
Goat, 86
whey, 87-88
God, 72-73, 93, 96
God force, 25-26, 31, 48, 53, 65, 93, 110
Goose, 110
Grains, 113-116
brown rice, 114-115
how to prepare, 115
millet, 114-116
rye, 114-115
wheat, 113-114, 116
yellow cornmeal, 114,-115
Grape juice, 103
Gravity, 51, 111
Gray, Robert, 40, 43-44
Great Salt Lake, 68
Green pepper, 79, 83
Grits, 27

H
Hair, 47, 53, 58, 61, 97
Halva foods, 103
Hand, 99, 107, 111
Happy and healthy, naturally..., 117-121

Harmony, 26, 31, 37, 42, 71-72, 95
Hate, 64
Hawthorn berry tea, 58
Head, 51, 77-78, 123
Headaches, 42
Healing crisis, 123, 124
Heart, 29, 37, 51, 55, 58, 77, 81, 103, 111-112
Heart attacks, 55
Hemorrhoids, 20
Hepatic flexure, 39
Herbal teas, 57-60
alfalfa, 59
comfrey, 58
cornsilk, 59
dandelion, 59
flaxseed, 42, 58
hawthorn berry, 58
horsetail (shavegrass), 59
how to prepare, 57
oat straw, 58
pau d'arco (taheebo), 59
peppermint, 58
red raspberry, 59
uva ursi, 59
Herbs, 17, 29-30, 42-43, 57, 79
Hering's law of cure, 123
healing crisis, 123-124
Herring, 110
High Desert® Honeybee PollenS™, 22
Hog, 109
Honey, 22, 50, 57, 88, 115
Honeybee, 21
Hormones, 61, 105
Horse, 58
Horsetail tea, 59
shavegrass tea, 59
Howard, Dr. A.B., 29
Human growth hormone (HGH), 46
Hydrochloric acid (HCl), 45-46, 86

I

Iceberg head lettuce, 83-84
Iced tea, 59
Ileo-cecal valve, 37, 39
Ileum, 37
Illness, 39, 51
Immune system, 59, 87, 105, 108
Indigestion, 46
Infections, 108
International Units (I.U.), 112
Iodine, 61-62
Ionic minerals, 69
Iron, 15, 20, 27, 30, 35, 59, 68, 83-84, 86
   black foods, 35, 83
Isaiah, 73
Isoleucine, 15
Israel, 88, 109
Itching, 77

J

Jarvis, Dr. D.C., 22
Jensen, Dr. Bernard, 16, 32-33, 35, 37, 39-42, 44-45, 51, 54, 61-64, 81, 84-87, 89-90, 97-100, 103, 111-114, 116, 123-124
Job, 72
Joints, 86
Joshua, 88

K

Kelp, 61
Kidney infections, 50
Kidneys, 37, 50, 59, 81, 100

L

Lactobacteria, 43
Laetrile, 114
Lamb, 110
Large intestine, 37, 39, 41-43, 58
Laws, 26, 31, 64, 93, 109-110
   balance, 31
   cleanliness, 109
   emotional, 31
   energy, 31
   harmony, 31
   love, 31, 64
   mental, 31
   nutritional, 31
   physical, 31
   spiritual, 31
Laxative, 20, 42, 53, 83
Lead, 73-74
Learn to love, 63-65
Lecithin, 20, 22, 90, 111-112
   cholesterol, 90, 111-112
   essential fatty acids, 112
Legs, 51, 95, 99
   "pumps" of the body, 51
Lemon, 57
Lettuce, 83-84
   bib, 83
   iceberg head, 83-84
   red leaf, 83
   romaine, 83
Leucine, 15
Leviticus, 109
"Life Energy," 106
Linoleic acid, 54
Linolenic acid, 54
Lipase, 45
Lips, 79
Liquid minerals, 67-69
Liver, 37, 39, 46, 48-49, 59
Lobster, 110
Loofah brush, 99
Love, 31, 63-65
Low blood carbohydrate, 50, 59, 98
Lubricant, 41, 54
Lucifer, 73
Lungs, 17, 21, 37, 100
Lymph nodes, 105
Lymphatic system, 41, 86, 100
Lymphocytes, 105

Index

Lysine, 15-16
   fights viruses, 16

M
Magnesium, 15-16, 20, 22, 30, 35, 41, 69, 114
Maker, 26, 71, 93, 110
Malt extract base, 97-98
Manganese, 20, 62, 68, 83
Manthei, Dr. Joseph, 17, 36, 59, 71, 74-75, 79, 93, 95-96, 101, 111
Manthei, Pamela S., 17, 27
Maple syrup, 50
Margarine, 80
Marine Minerals, 68-69
Meat, 109-110
   "koshering," 110
Menstruation, 59, 61
Metabolism, 49, 55, 61
Methionine, 15
   works with essential fatty acids, 15
Milk, 85-88, 113, 116
   allergies, 85-87, 113, 116
   cow, 85-88, 113, 116
   goat, 85-88, 113
Millet, 114-116
Min-Col, 71-75
   dinosaurs, 71-74
   usage guidelines, 74-75
Minerals, 15, 17-18, 27, 41, 48-49, 53, 61, 67-69, 71, 73, 75, 81, 83, 87, 93
Miscarriage, 20
Molecules, 31, 35, 47-48, 67-68
Moses, 88, 109
Mouth, 16, 50, 107
Mucus, 43, 85, 87, 99, 113
Muehling, Eldon C., 48
Muscles, 16, 41, 46, 51, 81, 93, 100-101, 111, 114
Muscular tissue, 101

N
Nails, 53, 58, 71, 97
Natural Ovens of Manitowac, Wisconsin, 54
NatureMost® Laboratories Inc., 77, 112
Nature's Sunshine Products, 20, 44, 46, 60, 98, 112
Neck, 99
Nerves, 35, 112
Nervous system, 53, 58, 87, 97, 101
Neurology, 101
New Testament, 109
Niacin, 77-78
   flush, 77-78
   usage guidelines, 78
Nutrient, 16, 22, 27, 35, 37, 54-55, 60, 77, 83, 87, 89-90, 93, 96-98, 111
Nutrilite®, 16
Nuts, 116

O
Oat straw tea, 58, 98
Oats, 58
Oil, 41, 55
   flaxseed, 55
Old Testament, 109-110
Olives, 83
Omega 3, 42, 54-55, 112
Omega 6, 42, 54, 112
Onion, 79, 83
Onion soup, 79-80
   how to prepare, 79-80
Orange pekoe tea, 59
Oregano, 17
Organs, 17, 37, 40, 42, 77, 99, 101, 105, 111
Oxygen, 52, 57-58, 111
Oysters, 110

P
Pain, 36

35 Practical Ways To Improve Your Health

Pancreas, 35, 105
Papain, 46
Papaya, 46
   papain, 46
Parotid glands, 46
Parsley, 79, 81
Pasteurized milk, 88
Pau d'arco tea, 59
   taheebo tea, 59
Peas, 83
Peppermint tea, 58
Pepsin, 45-46
Peristalsis, 42
pH, 45
Phenylalanine, 15
   anti-depressant, 15
Phosphate minerals, 71
   calcium, 71
   fluorine, 71
Phosphorus, 15, 22, 30, 87, 90
Photosynthesis, 35
Physiology, 101
Pigeons, 97
Pituitary gland, 46
Plantation Blackstrap Molasses, 28
Plants, 15, 19, 21, 35
   alfalfa, 15
   aloe vera, 19
   chlorophyll, 35
   honeybee, 21
Pollination, 21
   honeybee, 21
Pollutants, 47
Pores, 74
Pork, 110
Potassium, 15-16, 20, 22, 27, 30, 35, 41-42, 53, 81, 88, 93
Potato, 81
Potato peeling broth, 81-82, 124
   how to prepare, 81-82
Pregnancy, 20, 59, 74

Protease, 45
Protein, 45-46, 86, 113
Protein "splitters," 45
Prune, 42
   juice, 42
   steamed, 42
Psalms, 26
Psyllium, 43
Putrefactive bacteria, 43

R
Radishes, 83
Rain, 47-48
Rainbow-colored salads, 83-84
Raisins, 83
Rashes, 19
Raw goat's milk, 27, 85-88, 90, 113, 116
   allergy problems, 85-87, 113
   "feeds the whole body," 87, 113
   same makeup as mother's milk, 86, 113
Raw, whole, & pure, 41, 46, 83, 89-91, 97
Reagan, Ronald, 21-23
Reams, Dr. Carey, 20, 27, 49, 64, 71, 110, 113
Rectum, 39
Red leaf lettuce, 83
Red pepper, 29
Red raspberry tea, 59
"Reflex" action, 42
Rest, 93-94
Rheumatism, 81
Rhythm, 42, 52, 95-96
Rice bran syrup, 97-98
Rice polishings, 97
RNA, 46
Romaine lettuce, 83
Rose hips, 79
Royal, Penny C., 15, 29, 58

Index

Rutin, 22
Rye, 114-115

S
Salads, 18, 41, 54, 83-84
Saliva, 46
Salmon, 110
Salt, 61, 86
Salt water, 68, 110
Satan, 73
Scandinavian countries, 114
Sea kelp, 61
Seasonings, 17
Seawater, 68
Seaweed, 61-62
Seeds, 42, 53-54, 83, 103, 112
Sesame seed butter, 54, 103
   Westbrae Natural®, 103
Shavegrass tea, 59
   horsetail tea, 59
Shrimp, 110
Sigmoid colon, 39
Sigmoid flexure, 39
Silicon, 15, 42, 53, 58-59, 81, 97-98
Sinus conditions, 113
Skin, 19, 22, 41, 53, 58, 79, 97, 99-100
   "enlivened," 99
   "third" kidney, 100
Skin brush, 77, 99-100
Small intestine, 37, 58, 114
Sodium, 15-16, 20, 41, 69, 81, 86, 88
Sodium chloride, 86
Soft rock phosphate, 71, 73
Soups, 18, 30, 79-80
Soybean oil, 112
   essential fatty acids, 112
Specific gravity, 67-68
Spices, 17
Spinach, 83
Spinal adjustments, 101-102
Spine, 101

Spiritual, 25-26, 31, 65
Spleen, 37, 39, 105
Splenic flexure, 39
Spring water, 48
Sprouts, 83
Squash, 42, 83
Sterile, 22
Sternomanubrial joint, 106
Stitt, Dr. Paul, 54-55
Stomach, 29, 45-46, 58, 77, 86
   gas, 46
Stones, 59
Stool, 41-42, 54
   lubricant, 41-42, 54
Strength, 103, 105
Strokes, 22, 55
Sugar, 27, 42, 60, 103, 116
Sugar cane, 27, 89
Sugar level, 35
Sulphur, 15, 28, 30
Sunlight, 35
Supplements, 16, 30, 45, 53-55, 62, 67, 75, 98
Supreme Being, 25
Swine, 109

T
T cells, 105
Taheebo tea, 59
   pau d'arco tea, 59
Tahini foods, 103
Tannic acid, 59
   black tea, 59
   chocolate, 59
   iced teas, 59
   orange pekoe tea, 59
Taste buds, 50, 60, 88
Tea - see Herbal teas,
Tea strainers, 57
Teeth, 15, 71, 85, 87, 107
Tenney, Lousie, 29, 58-59
The President's Lunch™ Bar, 23

35 Practical Ways To Improve Your Health

Theobromine, 59
Thoughts, 25, 63-64
   negative, 63-64
Threonine, 15
Thymus gland, 105-108
   governs immune system, 105, 108
   "Life Energy," 106
   thump your thymus, 106-108
Thyroid gland, 61
   hyperactive, 61
   hypoactive, 61
   thyroxine, 61
Thyroxine, 61
Tissue, 42, 53, 100-101
Tomatoes, 83
Tongue, 27, 79, 107
Tooth decay, 47
Toxins, 37, 41, 43, 48-50, 100
Trace minerals, 15, 22, 27, 41, 67
Transverse colon, 39
Tryptophan, 15-16
   sleep aid, 16
Tuna, 110
Turkey, 103, 110

U
Ulcers, 15, 29
   peptic, 15
Unclean meats, 109, 110
   catfish, 110
   clams, 110
   duck, 110
   goose, 110
   lobster, 110
   oysters, 110
   pork, 110
   shrimp, 110
   tuna, 110
Undigested food, 37
Unpasteurized milk, 87-88
Unsaturated fatty acids, 53
Urine, 59
Uterus, 59
Uva ursi tea, 59

V
Vagus nervous system, 101
Valine, 15
Varicose veins, 112
Vegetables, 18, 27, 41, 49, 79, 83-84, 87, 116
Vegetarians, 87, 90
Villi, 114
Virus, 88
Vitamin
   A, 15, 22, 30, 35, 83
   B-complex, 15, 22, 30, 97
   B-3, 22, 77
   B-6, 22, 55
   B-17, 114
   C, 15, 22, 30, 79-80
   D, 15, 22
   E, 15, 22, 35, 103, 111-112
   F, 42, 53-54
   K, 15, 35
   P, 22
   U, 15
Vitamin A
   orange & yellow vegetables, 83
Vitamin B-3
   niacin, 77
Vitamin B-17
   laetrile, 114
Vitamin E
   d-Alpha Tocopherol, 112
   d-Alpha Tocopheryl Acetate, 112
   dl-Alpha Tocopheryl Acetate, 112
   "heart" vitamin, 111
Vitamin F
   essential fatty acids, 53
Vitamin K
   blood clotting, 15

Index

Vitamin P
   rutin, 22
Vitamin U
   peptic ulcers, 15

W
Walker, Dr. Norman W., 39
Walking, 51-52
Walking shoes, 52
Water, 27, 43, 46-50, 54, 57, 61, 68, 78, 88-89, 110, 115
Water distillers, 50
   stainless steel, 50
Wave set, 53
Wax beans, 83
Weight problems, 61
Westbrae Natural®, 103
Wheat, 113-114, 116
   allergies, 113, 116
   gluten content, 113
Wheat germ, 97-98
Whex®, 87
White blood cells, 105
White rice, 97
Whole brown rice, 98, 114-115
Whole grains, 80, 113-116
Whole wheat flour, 89, 113
Wounds, 58

Y
Yale University study, 114
Yeast, 97-98
Yellow cornmeal, 114-115

Z
Zinc, 20, 55

35 Practical Ways To Improve Your Health

Easy reading comes from difficult writing.
(variation of a quote by Robert Louis Stevenson)

ORDER FORM

Postal Orders: Real-Life Publications
8124 33rd Place North, Dept. B
Minneapolis, MN 55427-1921

Telephone Orders: (612) 544-5471

Please send me your book entitled: *35 PRACTICAL WAYS TO IMPROVE YOUR HEALTH* (allow 3 to 4 weeks time for delivery). I understand that I may return it to you for a full refund—at any time and for any reason, no questions asked.

Number of copies I am ordering _____ @ $9.95 each = $ _____

Minnesota residents please include appropriate
state sales tax (City of Mpls. pay 07%)   x 6.5% = $ _____

                                      Sub-Total = $ _____

ADD:
Shipping — $2.00 for the first book,
           $.75 for each additional book
           $3.50 per book for Air Mail   = $ _____

Enclosed is my: check ☐   M. O. ☐   **TOTAL** = $ _____
(make payable to "Real-Life Publications")

No cash, credit cards, or C.O.D.'s please.

- FOREIGN ORDERS: U.S. FUNDS ONLY, MONEY ORDER -

Prices subject to change without notice.

Mail book(s) to:

                          Date _____

Business Name: _____

Your Name: _____
                       (Please Print)

Address: _____

City: _____ State: _____ Zip: _____

Telephone #: (_____) _____